The Stand-Up Paddler's Guide to Southern California

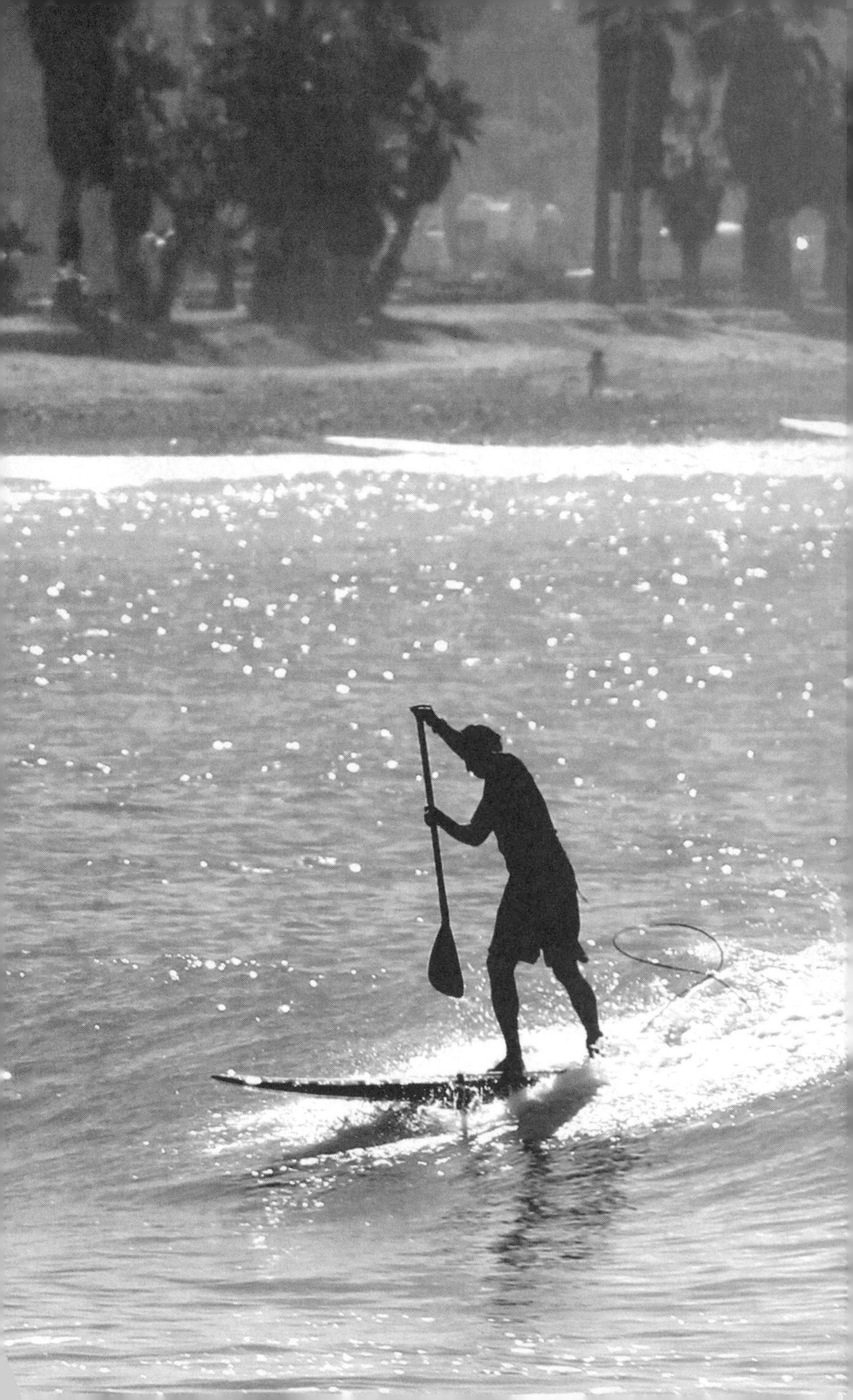

The Stand-Up Paddler's Guide to Southern California

Paddling, Surfing, Touring, Racing, and Yoga

David Womack

MENASHA RIDGE PRESS
Your Guide to the Outdoors Since 1982

The Stand-Up Paddler's Guide to Southern California

First edition, first printing

Editor: Lisa C. Bailey
Project editor: Ritchey Halphen
Cover photo: A.belloc (Own work) [CC-BY-SA-3.0], via Wikimedia Commons
Interior photos: David Womack except where noted
Maps: Steve Jones and David Womack
Cover design: Scott McGrew
Text design: Annie Long
Proofreader: Susan Cullen Anderson
Indexer: Sylvia Coates

Library of Congress Cataloging-in-Publication Data

Womack, David, 1963–
The stand-up paddler's guide to Southern California : paddling, surfing, touring, racing, and yoga / by David Womack. — First Edition.
pages cm
"Distributed by Publishers Group West"—T.p. verso.
ISBN 978-0-89732-481-6 — ISBN 0-89732-481-1 — ISBN 978-0-89732-482-3 (e-book)
1. Stand-up paddle surfing—California, Southern—Guidebooks. 2. California, Southern—Guidebooks. I. Title.
GV840.S68W6 2015
797.3'2097949—dc23
2015012277

Manufactured in the United States of America

Distributed by Publishers Group West

MENASHA RIDGE PRESS
An imprint of Keen Communications, LLC
PO Box 43673
Birmingham, AL 35243

Visit **menasharidge.com** for a complete listing of our books and for ordering information. Contact us at our website, at **facebook.com/menasharidge,** or at **twitter.com/menasharidge** with questions or comments. To find out more about who we are and what we're doing, visit our blog, **trekalong.com.**

Frontispiece: Catching a wave at Doheny State Beach (see page 179)

Disclaimer Although Menasha Ridge Press and David Womack have made every attempt to ensure that the information in this book is accurate at press time, they are not responsible for any loss, damage, injury, or inconvenience that may occur while using this book. You are responsible for your own safety and health in and around the ocean. Always check local conditions, and know your own limitations.

Table of Contents

Acknowledgments

FIRST AND FOREMOST, Keen Communications made this book possible. In particular I'd like to thank Tim Jackson, who believed in the project, was patient when chapters were late, and capably answered all my questions. Thanks also to project editor Ritchey Halphen for overseeing the completion of the book.

In a short timeline, it's impossible to find, explore, and paddle every single beach in Southern California. Thankfully, I was able to tap a few resources to make the process easier. The user forums on the Stand Up Zone website (**standupzone.com**) provided helpful insights to places I had never been. Many thanks to the Leo Carrillo sailboarders who gave me valuable tips about Malibu beaches. Thanks to Kenneth Rosenberg, who helped me navigate through La Jolla and Pacific Beach and taught me a thing or two about burritos. Matt Poth of 2 Stand Up Guys also provided helpful information about San Diego paddling locations. Mark Kubr convinced me to make a return trip to the South Bay, and I'm glad I did. I'm not a racer, but Kristin Thomas actually made me consider the prospect of racing SUPs. I'd like to thank her for her time, her insight, and her shared enthusiasm for the sport.

Thanks also to Izzy Tihanyi at Surf Diva, who provided some great action photos of paddlers and paddle surfers in and around La Jolla.

Finally, Joe Blair not only convinced me to ride a shorter board but also gave me insight into the board-making process, as well as some nice surfing tips and a bit of insider knowledge about Cardiff Reef. Joe is a knowledgeable shaper and an enthusiastic waterman. He will happily sell you a board, and then you'll be happy, too.

—*David Womack*

Introduction

SINCE YOU'RE ALREADY holding this book, you may not need the following encouragement, but here goes: If you haven't already begun to stand-up paddle, then you should start. If you've tried a stand-up paddleboard once, or even twice, and found it difficult, then you should try again. Truly. With the correct equipment, and maybe even a bit of instruction, just about everyone can enjoy the sport of stand-up paddling (SUP for short).

It makes sense that SUP is the fastest-growing water sport on the planet. Not only is it fun and a great way to get active, it provides an easy and effective means to experience the ocean—to get out on the water, to get a firsthand view of our scenic coastline. In Southern California, we have access to a large swath of the Pacific. Our beaches, harbors, and estuaries offer a variety of venues with a variety of conditions that are all, in their own way, perfect for this multifaceted sport. If you don't believe me, just ask the thousands of California SUP enthusiasts who are already out there paddling, racing, surfing, touring, and striking yoga poses.

For centuries, people have been paddling boats, canoes, and kayaks for the sake of commerce, travel, and adventure. Human-powered crafts tend to be some of the most basic and the most utilitarian boats on the water; they're also a great source of exercise.

SUP is a recent phenomenon—the natural evolution of the human-powered craft. By most accounts, it was introduced to California in 2004, and the first dedicated SUP shop didn't open its doors until 2007. Now, just a decade later, nearly every major beach city in Southern California has some sort of stand-up-paddle store. Across the Southland, there are outfits offering rentals and lessons as well as SUP fitness and yoga classes.

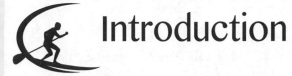

The stand-up paddleboard offers myriad possibilities. It's a great activity for men and women, young and old. Although it is an upstart sport, it's not a novelty—no more than bicycling is a novelty. There is much to do, to see, and to experience on a stand-up board, and although the basics of stand-up paddling can be learned in a day, experienced paddlers will continue to be challenged as they refine their techniques, try new SUP-related activities, and paddle to new far-flung locations.

Kayaking may be enjoyable, but stand-up paddling has added benefits. Being upright while paddling necessitates an extra level of muscle awareness. Balancing teaches us to use our core, strengthen our backs, and improve our posture. Standing up also provides a great vantage point to see above and below the water. While paddling across the water, SUPers can shift their focus between two distinct worlds—watching marine life, watching the coastline—while gliding gracefully toward the horizon.

Like surfing, stand-up paddling came to California from Hawaii. In the mid-1990s, big-wave surfers Laird Hamilton and Dave Kalama began paddling tandem surfboards with modified outrigger paddles. Eventually, they began shaping boards specifically for stand-up paddling. As SUP grew in popularity, Laird Hamilton in particular became its ambassador, pushing the limits on his own stand-up board while encouraging others to take up the sport.

Of course, Hamilton wasn't the first person to stand-up paddle; he just made it popular. From the 1950s to the 1990s, a group of local Waikiki surfers known as the Beach Boys (not the band) used paddles to push their boards into the Oahu beach's slow-moving waves. These Waikiki stand-up surfers may have drawn influence from outrigger canoes, or they may have been copying Duke Kahanamoku: Decades earlier, the surf pioneer was photographed standing and paddling a surf ski into waves at Waikiki. (One theory held that he surfed with a paddle to keep his camera dry, enabling him to photograph surfing tourists.) Even before the Duke, stand-up paddling may have been practiced in precolonial Hawaii. According to legend, Hawaiian chiefs, who apparently rode larger surfboards to signify royal largesse, used paddles to maneuver the bulky boards through the surf. Whether this legend is true is left to a few murky accounts of Hawaiian history, but the story is popular among SUP enthusiasts—and the reason the sport is sometimes referred to as "the sport of kings."

When SUP spread to the mainland, the possibilities of the sport quickly expanded. No longer just for elite athletes, stand-up paddling became accessible to nearly everyone. And as the popularity of the sport has grown, so has the number of SUP-related events: charity paddles, meet-up groups, and organized races. The SUP racing community is particularly strong in Southern California. Races are held year-round, with divisions for paddlers of all ages and abilities.

It's difficult to imagine Southern California without its beaches, which are essential to our lifestyle and recreation. That lifestyle now has a new outlet. And SUP makes every beach day a bit better. Stand up and take the opportunity to explore, to experience marine wildlife, to promote your fitness, and simply to forget about every problem that living a life on land offers us. The adventure merely begins at the shoreline.

This book serves as a guide to many of Southern California's finest paddling spots: harbors, beaches, and surf breaks. Whether you already have a board, plan to buy one, or expect to rent equipment, this book is designed to help you maximize your experience on the water.

How to Use This Book

ALTHOUGH THIS BOOK presents a cross-section of paddling locations in Southern California, it is by no means a complete list. With the right conditions, nearly every beach in the Southland can be a worthwhile location for stand-up paddling. In each chapter, I've provided helpful information about the local water conditions—the benefits and the difficulties associated with a particular venue. Of course, weather is far from constant, so be aware that conditions can vary.

For most locations, I purposely didn't outline specific paddle routes—merely preferred launch spots and destinations of interest. On any given day, numerous factors will determine where you will want to paddle. Weather, surf, and tides are frequent variables; crowds in and out of the water can be a factor too. Where possible and appropriate, I've listed multiple launch spots for paddling in a particular location. Beaches change, conditions change, and some days you just can't get a good parking spot.

Use this book as a guide, a starting point, but also be aware of current conditions. Before you go out, check the weather, check the wind, and, if appropriate, check the surf. At your disposal are plenty of resources for marine forecasts and current marine conditions. It's not only important to be safe, it's also important to maximize your experience. Make every day of paddling a great one.

Getting On Board, Part One: Knowing Your Gear

AT FIRST GLANCE, SUP gear seems pretty basic—you have a board and you have a paddle—but on closer inspection, you will learn that there are plenty of variables in the types of boards, and there are even different types of paddles. The process of winnowing down all your options may seem a bit overwhelming for a beginner. The best solution is to go out and paddle, try different boards, talk to your friends that paddle, and talk to the representatives at your local shop. But before you test the waters (or paddle them), you may need a bit of basic information.

How Much to Spend

ALTHOUGH THERE IS typically a direct relationship between cost and quality, many expensive boards may not be appropriate for all users—not everyone needs to drive a Ferrari, after all. Some big-box stores sell SUP boards at bargain prices; they'll get you out on the water, but they won't necessarily allow you to explore all the dimensions of the sport.

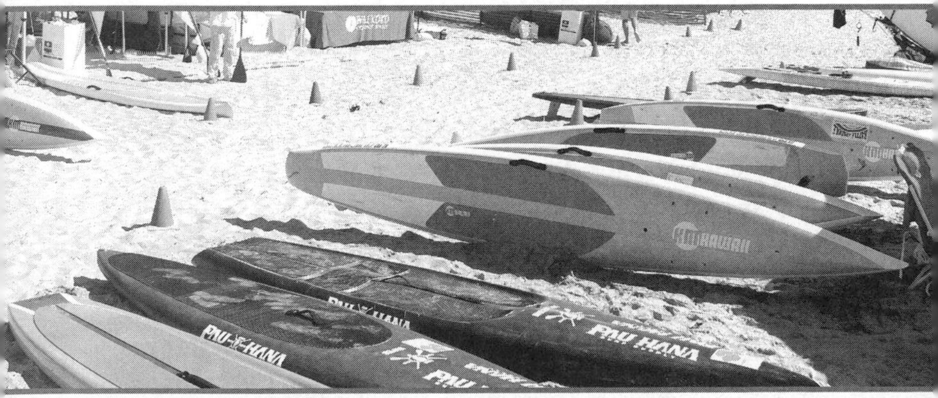

Racing boards lined up on the sand

Overall, it's important to be honest about your particular needs and expectations. Purchasing an SUP board can be a significant investment, so it's important to be smart. Buy a board that is comfortable for you, a board that is durable, and, if necessary, a board that will enable you to progress in the sport.

Renting Versus Buying

Renting is a great option, but if you plan on paddling frequently, it probably won't continue to be cost-effective. It also may not be as convenient: If you own your own board, you can paddle where you want, when you want. Of course, owning a board also means having to store the thing. There are some facilities near the water (typically at marinas) that provide board storage, but most board owners will be forced to store their own equipment. Thankfully, stand-up paddleboards are flat and easily slide under decks, can be shelved on the sides of garages, or can hang under awnings. A number of companies make board-specific racks that can easily be mounted to walls, ceilings, or overhangs. For those without adequate storage room indoors, there's always the option of purchasing a board bag. Even as the bag weathers, the board should remain in good shape.

As I've already mentioned, beginning paddlers should try different boards to determine their needs and preferences. First-time buyers may quickly outgrow their board, so renting, using a board for demonstration purposes, or borrowing one for an extended period—at least until you feel comfortable on the water—may be a smart option. This will help you get a feel for the sport and how much flotation you require (or will eventually require as you progress in the sport). Sometimes manufacturers hold demonstration days (demos) at the beach, where potential buyers are allowed to try various boards. Also, many shops have flexible demonstration plans—you pay a flat fee and get to try as many boards as you like until you find the one that's right for you. Dedicated SUP shops typically stock a greater variety of boards than on-site rental outfits. Many rental companies cater to tourists and stock only bulletproof (read: heavy) beginner boards.

Ultimately, whether you rent or buy will be determined by where, when, and how much you want to paddle. *Warning:* The sport can be addictive. You may find yourself buying multiple boards to satisfy all your paddling needs. Again, the best advice I can give is to be smart about what you buy: Purchase boards that you can grow into, are durable, and have proven designs.

Choosing the Correct Board

BUYING AN SUP board is a bit like buying a car: You have plenty of options to choose from—different materials, construction methods, and styles—at a wide range of prices. Beyond cost, a board's volume, shape, and construction are probably the most important considerations. For some buyers, however, other factors might also come into play—deck padding, cosmetic appeal, and whether the board fits in their garage or not.

Volume

Stand-up paddleboards are measured in feet and inches—length, width (at the wide point), and thickness. However, most large-production SUP brands also will list the volume of their boards in liters (particularly those brands that also make windsurfing boards, such as Bic, JP, Mistral, Naish, and Starboard). Beginner boards and touring boards can displace upwards of 200 liters, while some surf-specific SUP boards are rated at less than 100 liters.

The metric system tells us that 1 liter of displacement (volume) will support 1 kilogram of weight on the water, but just because your board floats you doesn't mean you'll be able to balance on it. For beginning paddlers, a general rule of thumb is at least 2 liters of board volume for every kilogram of rider weight. For example, if you weigh 175 pounds (roughly 80 kilograms), then you should be suited for a board with 160–180 liters of volume. Your level of athleticism, where you use the board, and how you use the board are important variables when determining necessary volume. For stand-up surfers in particular, progressing in the sport may necessitate going to a smaller board.

Local producers and shapers may not measure their boards by volume but instead may use the less-exacting measurement of board thickness to determine flotation. In this case, it's best to speak with someone at the shop to determine your specific needs. In general, 4.5–5.0 inches of thickness makes for a "floaty" board (depending on length, of course), 3.5–4.5 inches might be moderately floaty, and anything less will be best for smaller paddlers or advanced paddlers.

Lastly, not all 180-liter boards are created equal: The placement of the volume, the shape, and even the fins will affect the stability of the board. For larger riders, wider, rounder boards may be easier for balancing, but these are less efficient to paddle and don't track well in windy or choppy conditions. Longer, narrower boards paddle faster but aren't as stable. Larger fins will help with stability and tracking, but they make the board slower to turn. Ideally, every paddler should find his or her sweet spot—a board that paddles well enough, is stable enough, and is easy enough to maneuver.

Shape

SUP producers and enthusiasts can argue about the particulars of board shapes ad infinitum. Every shaper thinks his or her boards are the best, based on their specific use of rail design, rocker, volume distribution, and fin placement.

Details aside, a board's general shape is determined by its intended use or application:

≋ **Cruising boards or beginner boards** are typically long, fairly wide, and voluminous. They also have rounded tails and rounded noses. These boards are designed for an easy paddling experience, and although they may be heavy and difficult to maneuver in tight spaces, they are extremely stable on the water.

≋ **Racing boards** tend to be long and relatively narrow (12–14 feet long and generally less than 30 inches wide), with narrow noses and displacement hulls that effectively cut through the water. Although these boards possess moderate amounts of volume, they are designed for speed, not stability.

A Glossary of Board Shapes

Rails The edges of the board—more specifically, the point of transition from the bottom of the board to the side of the board. Rails can be rounded (soft) or steeply angled (sharp).

Nose The front of the board, which may have a rounded profile (spoon nose) or a narrow, pointy profile.

Tail The aft portion of the board, which can vary dramatically in width and shape. Beginner boards tend to have wide, rounded tails for stability; surfing SUP boards may have narrower pintails, sharply angled square tails, or even V-shaped swallowtails.

Rocker The amount of bend along the length of the board. Typically, rocker is most prevalent in the nose and the tail of the board. Nose rocker keeps the board from diving or "pearling" in waves or chop, while tail rocker typically makes the board looser and easier to turn. However, too much rocker results in less glide and therefore makes the board slower to paddle.

Outline The shape of the board as viewed from above, from nose to tail.

≋ Wider and more voluminous than racing boards, **touring boards** tend to have raked noses and displacement hulls. These boards also may have tie-downs for stowing gear.

≋ **Stand-up surfing boards** vary greatly in shape, but they tend to have less volume than other types; they also feature multiple fin setups. Some stand-up surfboards are shaped more like longboard surfboards, with straight long rails. Others are more oval-shaped—wide in the center and narrower at the tail. Those with round outlines generally turn more effectively in the surf but have less glide and tracking while paddling.

≋ **Hybrid boards** have enough volume for cruising, as well as narrower tails and multiple fin setups that aid in surfing.

≋ Lastly, **yoga-specific boards** tend to have plenty of volume for stability and softer deck pads to cushion hands and knees while doing poses. Paddling speed and maneuverability aren't as vital.

Construction

The majority of boards are made with foam blanks and then wrapped with fiberglass and sealed with epoxy resin. Although this may seem fairly straightforward, numerous variations come into play regarding the types of foam and fiberglass construction. Less-expensive boards may use lower-density foam and thin layers of fiberglass; this may result in a relatively light board that lacks durability. Boards made with lower-density foam may also be vulnerable to waterlogging—as soon as the outer skin is damaged, they should be removed from the water immediately. Higher-density foam blanks are often stronger and definitely more water-resistant, but they are also heavier.

Another process involves sandwiching low-density foam blanks between thin sheets of high-density foam core (like Divinycell) before adding layers of fiberglass. This adds to the board's structural integrity without adding too much weight. Race boards often use carbon fiber in order to make the them light and strong; these boards tend to be expensive because of the cost of the materials and the extra labor involved.

Many name-brand or production boards come with an application of Gel Coat, a veneer that adds cosmetic appeal and provides an extra layer of protection for the fiberglass. If the Gel Coat cracks or chips, the board should remain watertight, but the specific area of damage may be slightly more susceptible to dings and punctures.

Soft-Top Boards

Also constructed from foam blanks, these boards typically have a sheet of polycarbonate sandwiched onto the bottom and a layer of ethylene-vinyl acetate (EVA) foam wrapped over the entire deck. Soft-top SUP boards have the advantage of being virtually indestructible. Rental houses often use these boards. Unfortunately, soft-tops tend to be heavy, and some may absorb water—and therefore get even heavier—after prolonged use.

Inflatable Boards

These boards represent a fairly small part of the SUP market, but their design has improved remarkably over the last few years. Nearly every major manufacturer carries at least one inflatable SUP board in their lineup. The appeal of these boards is that they are easy to store, easy to carry, and certainly easy to travel with. Some inflatables are also fairly light, considering their relative volume and flotation. Inflatables are popular with whitewater stand-up paddlers because they can absorb blows from submerged rocks.

Components of the Board

Deck and Deck Pad The area on the board where you stand. A thicker deck pad makes for a comfortable ride but also adds weight to the board.

Carrying Handle Because SUP boards are wide, the handle allows riders to heft the board down to the water.

Leash Plug A small insert at the tail of the board. Typically a string is looped around the bar in the plug, and then the leash is attached to the string with Velcro.

Vent Plug A plastic stopper that threads into the deck of the board. The vent plug prevents delamination (separation of the fiberglass

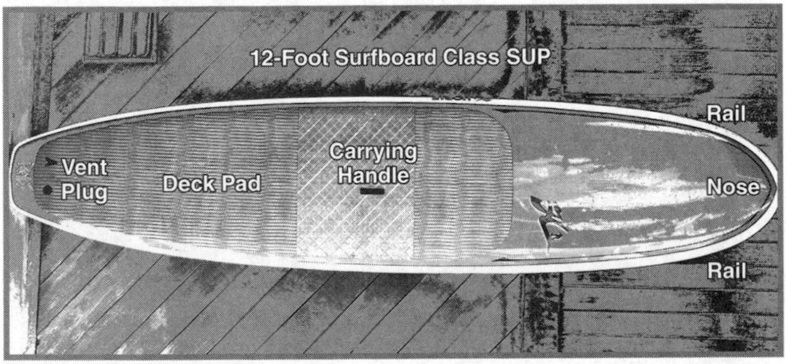

Your board, explained

from the foam blank), which may occur if the board is exposed to excessive heat or changes in pressure.

Release the vent plug when you plan to leave the board in a hot car or if you plan to take it on an airplane. Always be sure to retighten the vent plug before putting it back in the water. If your board is damaged and takes on water, release the vent plug while storing (and drying out) the waterlogged foam.

Fins Racing and touring boards typically have a single fin mounted in the center of the tail. Stand-up surfing boards and hybrid boards often have three fins. With the three-fin setup—sometimes called a thruster configuration—the center fin is larger and farther aft than the two opposing side fins. Other, particularly shorter, stand-up surfing boards may have two fins (a "twinzer"), four fins (quad), or five fins (single plus quad).

Fin Box Where the fin plugs in to the board. There are two primary types of fin boxes, with fins made specifically for each type:

The **American box** has a track that the back of the fin slides into. A screw is inserted through a hole in the front of the fin, then secured to a square, flat nut, also in the track of the fin box. The American box allows for adjustable fin placement (fore and aft) and is typically used in single-fin boards and for the center fin in three- or five-fin setups.

First developed in Australia, **FCS (fin-control system) boxes** do not allow adjustment and use an Allen wrench to secure the fin. These boxes are typically used for the board's smaller side fins.

Paddles

SUP PADDLES HAVE three major components: the **blade,** the **shaft,** and the **T-handle.** The **elbow,** between the shaft and the blade, gives the blade a forward cant. The T-handle inserts into the top end of the shaft, allowing the user to place one hand over the top of the shaft while paddling.

The overall length of the paddle is an important consideration. Some paddle manufacturers have detailed charts for sizing. As a general guideline, the entire length of the paddle should be about 6–10 inches longer than the height of the paddler. (Because of arm length, shorter paddlers will need less overage than taller paddlers). Some variables when considering paddle length include board thickness, the amount of extension in one's paddle stroke, and the conditions where you're paddling.

Because they bend their knees more, stand-up surfers tend to use slightly shorter paddles. Every paddler will probably need a bit of time on the water before determining his or her ideal paddle length. Typically, rental houses and shops have adjustable paddles on hand so users can test out different lengths.

Blade size is another important consideration when racing and touring. Large blades push more water, but they require more effort to do so. The easiest comparison is to gears on a bike—you can go faster in a big gear, but that also requires more energy. The nuances of blade shape and size may not be as important for casual users. Most beginning SUPers will use similarly styled paddles; however, smaller paddlers may want to use a smaller blade. Also, because the paddle also aids in balancing on the board, a larger blade may improve the rider's stability.

Most paddles are made from aluminum, fiberglass, or carbon fiber (wood is less commonly used). Aluminum paddles are the least expensive and probably the most prone to breaking. The metal also tends to corrode after multiple exposures to salt water. Carbon fiber is very light and strong, but it also makes for an expensive paddle. Good fiberglass and carbon-fiber paddles should flex under stress—and therefore be less prone to breaking. To test a paddle's flex characteristics, place the blade on the ground facing forward. Hold the T-grip in your outside hand, then use your other hand to put downward pressure on the shaft. With a moderate amount of force, the paddle should bend around the elbow and then quickly retract when the force is lifted.

Accessories

Leashes

Definitely a requirement in the surf and often advisable when paddling in the open ocean, a leash keeps the board tethered to the rider. Most leashes have a cuff that attaches to the rider's ankle; other leashes have a cuff that attaches below the knee. There are also coiled leashes that retract (like a telephone cord), reducing the amount of drag in the water—particularly helpful when paddling through kelp—and also lowering the chance that the cord will become tangled around the rider's leg or pinched beneath his or her heel.

A leash should be at least as long as the accompanying board. I recommend using an SUP-specific leash, which is stronger and tends to have a quick-release system, rather than a standard-issue surfboard leash. A quick release is particularly important when paddling near reefs and kelp—if the leash becomes snagged, the rider can become trapped near breaking waves or tidal surges.

One important safety note: *Never put your finger in the loop that attaches the leash to the leash plug.* Grabbing the SUP board in this manner may be tempting when you're in the water and the board is floating away from you, but it can result in serious injury.

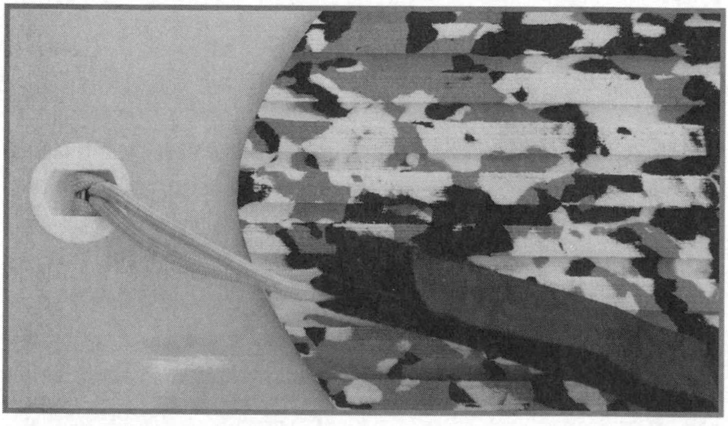

Leash plug with leash attached

Personal Flotation Devices (PFDs)

IN CALIFORNIA, SUP boards are designated as vessels and therefore subject to certain boating laws. Technically, all paddlers are required to wear or carry life vests. In practice, this rule is rarely enforced (the exception may be in certain harbors). Rental outfits typically provide paddlers with PFDs as a matter of safety and also to limit the company's exposure to legal indemnity.

For competent swimmers, PFDs probably aren't necessary; in fact, most SUPers never use them. But in case of an unexpected calamity, a PFD can save your life. For those who want the extra protection, there are life vests designed specifically for stand-up paddling.

Clothing and Wet Suits

In the summer months, when the water is moderately warm, most paddlers will need only to wear a swimsuit or a rash guard made from Lycra or another quick-drying material. When the water and the air are colder—and particularly if you plan on getting wet—you may find it necessary to wear a neoprene wet suit. Some wet-suit companies make SUP-specific products, including neoprene tops (or hybrid tops that are part neoprene and part Lycra), vests, and long johns–style suits.

Wearing a hat is often a good idea for sun protection. If you're expecting to get wet, note that a few types of surf hats are available. They're made of quick-drying material and have a chin strap that helps keep the brim secure on your head.

Booties

Where your feet are concerned, not all ocean beaches are created equal. Rocky shorelines can be uncomfortable underfoot, and even smooth rocks can become problematic when they're picked up and slammed on your toes by the shore break.

Paddlers with sensitive feet may consider wearing neoprene booties. The primary disadvantage of booties is that they make it harder to feel the board—the bottoms of your feet are your eyes when it comes to balancing, so try to find booties that are designed for surfing, which have a more natural feel on the board.

Surf booties vary in thickness; some are designed for warmth as well as protection. (Thinner surf booties are sometimes called reef socks.)

As an alternative to booties, you might try wearing plastic or rubber shoes into the water, then attaching those shoes to yourself while paddling. It may seem inelegant, but it will effectively protect your feet.

Hydration Packs

Drinking water is important when racing, training, or touring. Thankfully, there are hydration packs made specifically for SUP. The best packs are made with quick-drying material and have clips or lanyards that allow for easy and constant access to the drinking valve.

Getting On Board, Part Two: Launching and Paddling

Driving with Your Board

STAND-UP PADDLEBOARDS ARE big, so transporting them on your car requires some planning. If you own a standard car, you will most likely need roof racks. If your car doesn't have factory racks, several brands of aftermarket racks are available. The best systems have specific fittings for different models of cars, making installation relatively easy. Once you have the racks in place, use tie-down straps to secure the board. (I prefer the buckle-style straps sold in surf shops over the ratchet-style straps sold in hardware stores.) It's smart to put a couple of twists in the span where the straps reach across the surface of the board; this will keep the straps from vibrating when the car is traveling at speed.

I prefer to place the board on the rack with the nose forward and the fin facing skyward. To me, this seems natural and aerodynamic. Some safety guides suggest putting the board tail forward in order to reduce the risk of the board slipping out of the straps, the theory being that the fins will catch on the straps. My experience is that as long as the straps are rigid, the board won't slip. Never use stretchy tie-downs like bungee cords, and always make sure your straps are in good order—the material should not be weathered or frayed, and the buckles should effectively lock and hold the straps in place.

They're not the best option, but soft racks or temporary racks are sometimes necessary. In this case, you should loop an extra safety strap over the roof, pulling the ends through the two opposing side windows; the closed loop should then be pulled tightly and secured inside the car. The downside of this precautionary measure is that you won't be able to open two of your car doors while the strap is in place, but it will protect your board from launching off your car.

Carrying Your Board

STAND-UP PADDLEBOARDS TYPICALLY weigh no more than a couple bags of groceries; on the other hand, they're bulky and often difficult to carry. Fortunately, most modern SUP boards have an indented carrying handle, enabling you to hold the board to your side, like an oversize suitcase. If this method proves difficult—as it may in tight spaces such as crowded walkways and steep staircases—you may want to carry the board on your head, holding a rail in each hand. Another method is to lift the board from the bottom and balance one rail of the board in the crux of your elbow; the deck of the board will then lean against the side of your head, forming a triangle between your outstretched arm, the board, and your head. If the board is simply too big, or these methods seem daunting, then it might be a good idea to carry the board (or boards) in tandem with your paddling buddy.

The last option is to use a carrying sling, several brands of which are available online. Carrying slings typically involve two buckled straps that secure the board and an attached loop that goes over the rider's shoulder. A simple and effective homemade sling can be made with a tie-down strap. All you have to do is make a secure loop and slide it over the nose of the board until the loop is roughly perpendicular with the board's carrying handle. Once you get the loop to the correct size, pick up the board and lift the strap over your head and shoulder. If you're carrying the board in your right hand, the loop will go under your board, across your chest, in front of your left shoulder, and then behind your neck and right shoulder. Put your right hand in the carrying handle to stabilize the board.

Be aware when carrying an SUP board in breezy conditions—the surface of the board acts like a sail and may make it difficult to control the board or keep it in line with your body. Always try to keep the nose of the board facing either directly into the wind or directly away from it.

SUP Fundamentals

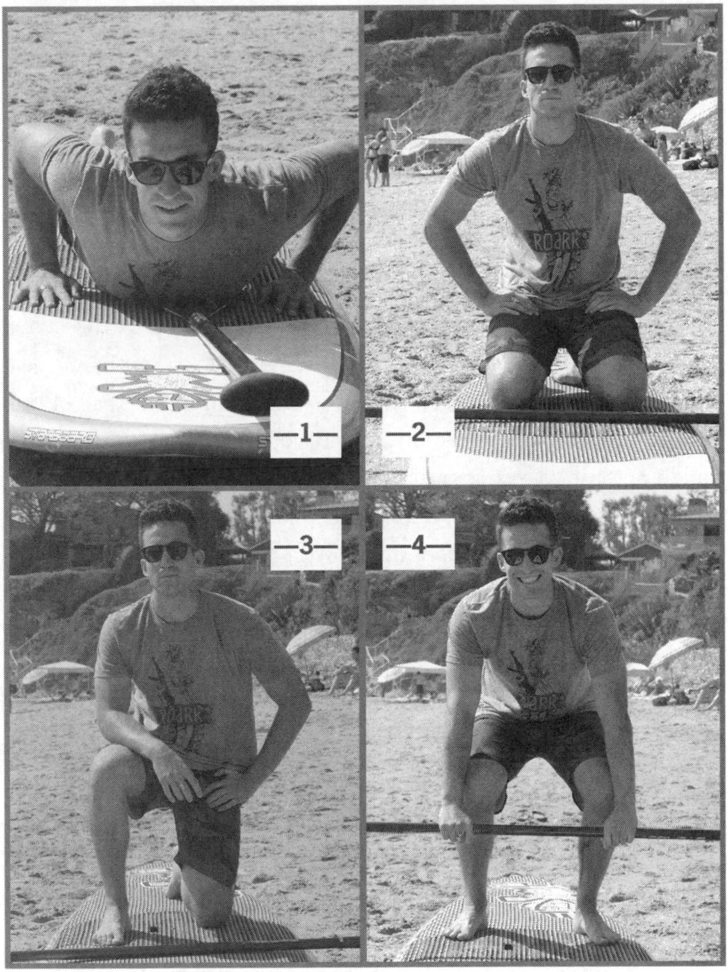

1 *Prone position with paddle secured under chest.*

2 *Kneeling position, with paddle lying across the board.*

3 *Preparing to stand, with one knee forward.*

4 *Feet side by side, knees bent. The next step is to get the paddle in the water.*

Standing on Your Board

ALTHOUGH STANDING UP on the board may seem daunting at first, this critical step can be mastered fairly quickly. Certainly having a stable board and calm conditions will make it easier to get on your feet, but external factors aside, being focused and confident will make the transition less difficult.

Before you attempt to stand, make sure you feel balanced and comfortable on the board—there's no rush. When you're ready, begin by placing the paddle across the board in front of you. Then pull one leg forward and plant that foot firmly onto the deck of the board, approximately in line with the carrying handle. Plant your hands near the paddle and pull your second leg forward, planting the ball of that foot parallel to, and comfortably behind, your front foot. Then grab the paddle and use your core muscles to help pull yourself upright.

As you stand, place your paddle blade in the water for stability, then pull your second foot in line with the first. Eventually, as you become more comfortable on the board, you should be able to make the transition quickly and fluidly. As you gain confidence, you may even be able to simply plant your hands and jump, feet forward, into the standing position, similar to the motion you'd use to do a jackknife off a diving board: Bend at the hips, and use your core to spring your legs forward. Popping up quickly and efficiently is essential when riding less stable boards or when going out in bumpy conditions. Regardless of the conditions, it's always important to move confidently and decisively. You shouldn't rush yourself, but hesitating midtransition is rarely beneficial. Always keep your legs firm, engage your core, and, when necessary, dig the paddle into the water for balance.

Balancing on Your Board

YOUR POSTURE AND position on the board are fundamental to your success as a paddler. Ideally, your feet should be shoulder-width apart, roughly on either side of the carrying handle. Imagine that each of your feet has four points of contact: the big-toe mound, the

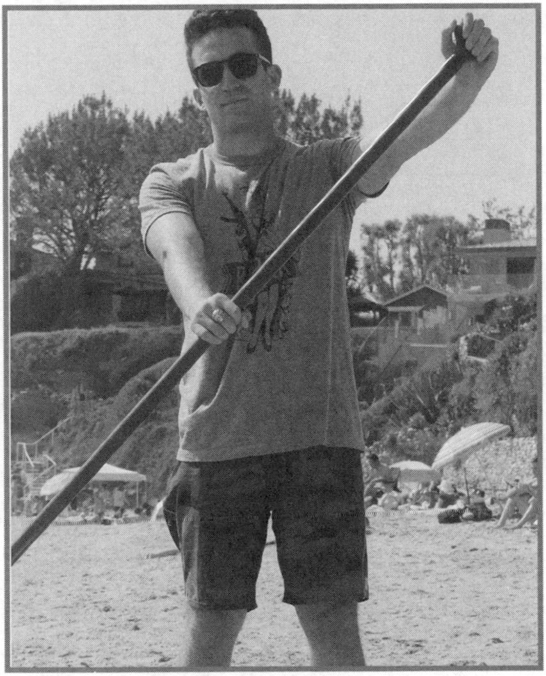

Standing up with the paddle in place

pinky-toe mound, the inside of the heel, and the outside of the heel. Try to weight each of these points equally on the board. Isometrically pull your shins together and put a slight bend in your knees. This will enable you to keep your hips fluid, which is important since you will be constantly adjusting to the movement and tilt of the board.

Contract the muscles just below your navel to engage your core while keeping your chest open, your torso upright, and your gaze toward the horizon. (One mistake that beginners make is constantly looking down at their feet. This has several disadvantages—it means you can't see where you are going, it affects your posture and makes you less stable, and it reduces the length and efficiency of your paddle stroke.) As much as possible, try to keep the paddle in contact with the water. If you become unsteady, bend your knees to lower your center of gravity.

For some riders, it may be beneficial to keep one foot slightly behind the other—a variation of their surf stance. This is perfectly acceptable; the staggered stance is used frequently by racers and by stand-up surfers when paddling over waves. For cruising and touring, however, you'll eventually be more comfortable with your feet side by side. If you do fall in the water, it's not a big deal. For most people, falling is part of the learning process. Just be sure not to fall on your board or on your paddle. If you lose your balance, simply bend your knees and lean away from the board, keeping the paddle at arm's length.

Holding the Paddle

THE MOST COMMON mistake beginners make is to hold the paddle backward. Although it may seem counterintuitive at first, the paddle has a forward cant. When you hold the paddle correctly, the blade should be angled away from the plane of your body and toward the front of the board.

Online Instructional Resources

If you're a visual person, you'll be happy to know that a wealth of information exists on the web to help you with basics such as standing and balancing. The following YouTube videos can help get you started.

This video demonstrates and explains basic SUP techniques for those who are new to the sport: **tinyurl.com/supbasics**

This video is designed to teach beginners the fundamentals, or "Golden Rules," of paddling and turning: **tinyurl.com/supgoldenrules**

The first video on this shows and explains paddling technique, provides a quick overview of several aspects of the sport, and includes a quick primer on paddle design and sizing: **quickbladepaddles.com/video/how-to-sup**

Finally, this video shows how to efficiently and effectively get back on your board if you fall off: **tinyurl.com/supgettingup**

The fingers of your top hand should be wrapped over the top of the T-handle, and your other hand should grip the paddle shaft comfortably around the level of your stomach. Your elbows should be slightly bent and your shoulders square to the front of your board.

Paddling

START IN A comfortable and stable stance, holding the paddle as described above. If your right hand is over the T-handle and your left hand on the shaft, then you'll want to begin by paddling on the left side of the board. Keeping your legs steady, initiate the stroke by slightly rotating your right hip and right shoulder. As you reach forward, the paddle will make contact with the water. Plunge the blade completely into the water before drawing the paddle back. Once the blade reaches the plane of your feet, twist your top hand slightly to release the paddle from the water.

When the blade has cleared the waterline, you're ready to make another stroke. Be sure to draw the paddle back parallel to the centerline of the board. Don't use your arms to paddle—your elbows should begin slightly bent and should remain somewhat rigid for the entire stroke. You will be able to paddle farther and more effectively when you draw power from the strong muscles in your torso and your core.

To maintain a straight course, you'll have to alternate sides with the paddle. After four to five strokes on the left side, take your right hand off the top of the paddle and place it on the shaft just below your left hand. As you move the paddle blade over the deck of the board, place your left hand over the T-handle. Now you're ready to start paddling on the right side. The paddle switch may feel cumbersome at first, but it's an essential skill for all aspects of the sport. Some guides suggest that beginners keep the same hold and twist the paddle across their bodies when necessary. I don't recommend this, however, because the cross-paddle is awkward and rather ineffective.

If you're having difficulty switching from hand to hand with your paddle, then practice the technique on land. While standing on a chair—so you have proper clearance for the paddle blade—take one stroke, switch hands, take another stroke, switch hands, and repeat until the transition becomes easy and fluid.

Key Paddling Points

1. Make sure the blade is completely in the water before you begin to pull the paddle back.
2. Don't use your arms—rely on the strong muscles in your core, your middle- and lower-back muscles, and your torso.
3. Don't draw the paddle too far back. Release the blade from the water as it comes in line with your feet.
4. Twist the paddle slightly before releasing the blade from the water.

Ideally, you want to maintain a stable position as you paddle, keeping the board level to the surface of the water. The more the board dips and yaws, the less efficiently it will move across the water. Additionally, the paddle should enter the water with minimal splash—think of an Olympic diver—and exit the water with minimal effort.

Launching

BEGINNERS WILL DEFINITELY find it easiest to launch in calm and protected waterways such as marinas or lagoons. Many marinas have gently sloped beaches or boat launches that make the transition from land to water fairly simple.

When launching in calm conditions, carry the board to the shoreline and place it in the water directly in front of you; then lay the paddle across the board a few inches in front of the carrying handle. Approaching from the side, carefully climb onto the board, placing your knees on either side of the handle. As soon as you're on the board, grab the paddle and make a stroke to get the board moving. Once the board is in motion, it will immediately become more stable. As you improve at launching, you should be able to push off a bit from the shore, putting the board in motion as you hop onto the deck.

Launching in the surf requires a different strategy and a more careful study of the conditions. Tidal surges and waves, particularly those breaking close to shore, present certain risks for SUPers (as well as nearby swimmers). However, there are safe and effective ways to launch your board in most conditions.

The first thing you should do when arriving at the beach is to look for a relatively calm stretch along the shore. If you find crowds of swimmers in your preferred launch area, you may need to negotiate with them to get a bit of space. At some beaches, the lifeguards are willing to assist, getting swimmers to move safely aside.

Before you enter the water, watch the surf for a while and assess the conditions. Waves typically come in sets that, depending on the swell, can be as much as 15 minutes apart. If you're unsure, consult with the lifeguard before heading out.

Once you've determined your launch area and the safety of the conditions, approach the shoreline with your board in one hand and the paddle in the other. If you're using a leash, the cuff should already be attached to your leg. Wade into the shallow water, holding the board above the tidal surge. Look out onto the water, past the breaking waves to see if there are more swells approaching. Patience is key. When it appears there are no incoming waves, walk the board farther out—deep enough for the fins to clear—and place it in the water beside you. Always keep the nose of the board facing toward the incoming surf, and never stand between the board and the shore, because an incoming wave could knock the board toward shore and directly into you. Once the board is in the water, climb onto it quickly. Beginners may want to paddle on their knees to get through the surf. Make short, quick paddles to get the board moving; again, keep the nose of the board facing directly toward the incoming surf.

Your board is big, and when powered by breaking waves, it can injure other water users. Even if you're using a leash, the far end of the board may drag 20–25 feet behind you. Never assume that swimmers understand the inherent dangers of a loose board in the surf.

To reiterate:

Be careful. Always assure your own safety and the safety of others when launching your board.

Be patient. Always wait for an interval of small surf before paddling out.

Be decisive. When there are no waves on the horizon, get on the board and quickly paddle outside of the surf zone.

Turning

PERHAPS THE EASIEST way to turn an SUP board is to continually paddle on one side. If you only paddle only on the right side, for instance, the board will turn left and eventually come about. This generally results in a slow, wide-arcing turn, but you can speed things along by paddling farther away from the side of the board, drawing the blade in the direction opposite that in which you are turning.

To make turns in tighter spaces—particularly if you don't want to move forward while coming about—you can back-paddle: Rotate the paddle blade backward and place it in the water at or behind your feet; then make a few quick back paddles, drawing the blade in short strokes toward the nose of the board. Once you've initiated the turn, make a couple of quick forward draws on the other side of the board. Then continue to alternate sides as necessary.

If you lack the arm strength to back-paddle, you can lever the paddle off your hip, using your body as a fulcrum to initiate the reverse stroke. The faster you move forward before you begin the back paddle, the more force you'll need to initiate the stroke.

The pivot turn is the quickest way to come about. This maneuver requires a bit of skill and balance, but it's an essential tool for racing and stand-up surfing—and a fun trick for everyone to try. Begin the turn by moving one foot toward the back of the board. As the tail sinks, bend your front knee and lean slightly forward. If your left knee is in front, you'll find it easiest to turn your torso slightly to the right and make quick, arcing paddle strokes, drawing away from the right rail (turning the board left). The board should pivot on the tail. Once it comes about, pull your back foot forward again, keeping the paddle blade in the water for stability.

Stopping

AS DESCRIBED PREVIOUSLY, back-paddling is also an effective way to stop the board. Just remember that when you initiate the stroke, the board also will turn in the direction of the paddle. If you want to stop without turning, alternate backstrokes on either side.

Another way to stop the board is to step one foot back and sink the tail. This method works well when the board is gliding on a wave or swell, but you should know your ability and use caution. If you step back and fall off the tail, the board will shoot forward—probably directly into the obstacle you intended to avoid.

Landing

LANDING ALONG PROTECTED shores requires little explanation. The main thing is to be careful not to damage your fins when you're approaching shallow water. If you can't see the bottom, it's typically best to drop to your knees before stepping off the board—you don't want to end your enjoyable paddling experience with a foot injury.

Landing at a dock may require a bit of jockeying and positioning. Use the above techniques for turning and stopping to make sure you don't damage your board. If the deck of the landing area is close to the waterline, you may be able to step directly off your board and onto the dock. If the landing deck is a few feet above the water, then use your hands to pull yourself alongside the dock. Place your paddle in a safe place, and then sit on the dock while keeping your feet firmly planted on the board (you don't want your board to float away). Eventually, you should be able to climb up on the dock and retrieve your board. If this proves difficult—for example, in rare cases when the dock is several feet above the water level—then use a leash to retrieve the board from the water.

When landing in the surf, you should use the same level of caution you would when going out through the waves. As you approach the surf zone, paddle to a section of shore that is clear of swimmers and waders. If there is no open space, signal to people in the water and let them know of your intention to land.

It never hurts to be patient. Keep your eyes on the horizon and wait for a relatively flat spell. When things looks safe, paddle quickly to the shore. It's usually best to paddle at a slight angle to the shoreline so you can see if waves are approaching behind you. (Don't overdo the angle, because the board could be broadsided by incoming waves. Also, your ability to look behind you while paddling will improve as you spend more time on the board.) You should try to calculate your approach to shore, following safely behind a small wave and then getting off the board as soon as the wave breaks in front of you. If you're in the surf zone and you feel yourself getting pulled backward, this means that a wave is forming behind you. Dismount before the wave reaches your board—the shore break is probably too steep to negotiate on an SUP board.

Some paddlers prefer to knee-paddle when they approach the shore. Whether on knees or feet, you need to effectively time your approach to the shore. Wait out the waves, then be decisive when you catch a lull in the surf. Always be aware of submerged rocks that could damage your fin or board. Paddle to the shore with the board angled away from the breaking waves. When you reach a shallow spot to dismount, step off, then quickly grab the board and carry it beyond the tide line. This is another skill that will improve with practice. As a beginner, simply avoid large surf and crowds of people, and never put yourself between the board and the shoreline.

Paddling in Wind and Chop

YOU SHOULD DEFINITELY master the basics of paddling before venturing out in rough conditions. If you're trying to learn SUP, then wind and chop will make the process frustrating. Even experienced paddlers will choose calm days over windy ones, but sometimes the weather simply doesn't cooperate.

At many Southern California beaches, the wind accelerates in the afternoon—a light breeze may turn into a stiff breeze while you are out on the water. For this reason, I almost always recommend a paddling course that begins windward and returns downwind. Once you reach your destination, the hard work will be over and the trip home will require much less effort.

Not all boards are created equal. Those with longer and narrower profiles, or ones with displacement hulls, have the best upwind performance. Depending on your board, and the strength of the wind, it may be necessary to zigzag upwind (tacking like a sailboat). To keep the board on track, you may need to switch paddle sides with greater frequency. Also, use short, quick paddle strokes and paddle close to—or even under—the rail of the board.

Turning the board may be difficult in choppy conditions. Again use short, quick strokes. Keeping the blade of the paddle in contact with the water will help with stability. As the board tilts and dips, maintain a deep bend in your knees, using your legs like shock absorbers. Try to keep a bit more pressure on the windward rail. If the underside of the board is exposed to the breeze, it may lift a bit out of the water, making the board quite unstable.

When paddling downwind, it may be necessary to stand a bit farther back on the board. This will keep the nose of the board riding higher and allow you to ride down the chop without "pearling," or planting the nose under the surface of the water. If the chop is fairly large, you may not be able to paddle straight to weather. Instead, angle back and forth to avoid pearling in the swells. The board will definitely be traveling faster when you head downwind. Be careful of kelp or other floating snags that may bring you to a sudden stop. If you're paddling downwind in open water, you should consider wearing a leash—getting separated from your board can be both dangerous and expensive.

Coastal Weather and Water Conditions

Weather Overview

PARTLY CLOUDY IN THE MORNING AND CLEARING IN THE AFTERNOON—this is the mantra for many Southern California meteorologists. Steve Martin parodied this phenomenon in the 1991 film *L.A. Story.* His character, Harris K. Telemacher, an eccentric TV weatherman, starts pre-taping his weather reports, betting on never-changing weather patterns. His career comes to a crashing halt after it unexpectedly rains one day. Oh, the horror.

Stuck in the gap between the cool water of the Pacific Ocean and the arid Mojave Desert, Southern California enjoys fairly mild weather year-round. Yes, there are Pacific storms that sweep down and bring rain, wind, and the accompanying havoc on the freeways, but these events are infrequent. Los Angeles averages only about 30 rainy and drizzly days per year, most of those concentrated in January, February, and March. Even in the midst of winter, there are beautiful sunny days. The water is colder in winter—about 8°–10°F cooler than summer temps—but on warm, clear January afternoons, surface conditions can be ideal for paddling.

In the spring and early summer, the coastal areas of Southern California are often covered in a dense marine layer. The condition, known as "May gray" or "June gloom," is created by the cool band of water that lies just off the coast. As our weather mantra indicates, the marine layer tends to draw back as the sun warms the land. For beachgoers, it's always a matter of how far it will draw back: Some days it can be perfectly sunny just blocks from the beach but remain damp and gloomy over the sand and water. If you're driving from inland hoping for sunny weather at the beach, it's always best to check an updated weather report or look at one of the local beach cams.

Here are the monthly averages for air temperature and precipitation as recorded at the Santa Monica pier (an aggregate of data collected from 1948 to 2005). The chart illustrates the temperate nature of Southern California's coastal climate; of course, daily temperatures may vary greatly from the mean.

Average Maximum Temperature					
Jan	**Feb**	**Mar**	**Apr**	**May**	**Jun**
63.9° F	63.5° F	63.0° F	63.9° F	64.8° F	67.3° F
Jul	**Aug**	**Sep**	**Oct**	**Nov**	**Dec**
70.3° F	71.3° F	71.5° F	70.0° F	67.8° F	64.7° F
Annual Average Maximum Temperature **66.8° F**					
Average Minimum Temperature					
Jan	**Feb**	**Mar**	**Apr**	**May**	**Jun**
49.6° F	50.3° F	51.2° F	53.2° F	55.8° F	58.7° F
Jul	**Aug**	**Sep**	**Oct**	**Nov**	**Dec**
61.4° F	62.5° F	61.7° F	58.5° F	53.8° F	50.0° F
Annual Average Minimum Temperature **55.6° F**					
Average Total Precipitation					
Jan	**Feb**	**Mar**	**Apr**	**May**	**Jun**
2.98 in.	3.04	1.94 in.	0.79 in.	0.20 in.	0.03 in.
Jul	**Aug**	**Sep**	**Oct**	**Nov**	**Dec**
0.02 in.	0.10 in.	0.13 in.	0.32 in.	1.46 in.	1.87 in.
Annual Average Total Precipitation **12.87 inches**					

Source: *Western Regional Climate Center*

Wind

FOR PADDLERS, WIND is the most critical weather element. Plenty of nice beach days evolve into poor paddling days when the afternoon sea breezes fill in. The prevailing coastal winds in Southern California are westerly, and these tend to ramp up in the afternoon. As the inland valleys heat up, a pressure gradient develops and the cooler, heavier ocean air rushes inland. The effect can be intensified by certain prominent landmasses. The afternoon sea breezes often accelerate along the near-shore coastal range between Point Mugu and Point Dume. Winds also funnel around the Palos Verdes Peninsula, creating breezy afternoon conditions from Cabrillo Beach in San Pedro down to Huntington Beach. In contrast, Santa Barbara, southern Orange County, and San Diego typically have less-prevalent afternoon winds.

Sometimes the Southern California waters will be chopped up by early-morning winds blowing out of the south or southeast—a phenomenon local surfers refer to as "morning sickness." It typically occurs when there are strong northwest winds pushing down from the central coast. These winds rush by Point Conception and then eddy counterclockwise around the Channel Islands. (Sometimes Los Angeles meteorologists refer to the occurrence as a "Catalina eddy.") As the winds bend southward, they typically also bring cool, cloudy conditions to the coast. When the eddy is strong, it will last all day, but particularly in the summer months, the condition often dissipates in the afternoon, allowing for the return of the prevailing westerlies.

The most famous winds in Southern California are the Santa Anas—the dry, dusty, and often destructive winds that typically blow in the fall and early winter. The strong gusts originate over the desert and reach great velocities in the inland valleys, but they often peter out before making it to the coast. Many Santa Ana days are perfect paddling days, but when Santa Anas do reach the beach, they blow directly offshore and have the potential to push paddlers out to sea. During Santa Ana events, always be careful when SUPing near canyon mouths. The offshore winds also tend to intensify in the evening and morning hours. Even though they bring warm midday temperatures, Santa Ana days may turn abruptly cooler as the sun goes down.

Northwest winds are the least common but often strongest winds along the coastal waters of Southern California. These events often occur in the wake of storms or fast-moving low-pressure systems. As the cloud masses pass by, northwesterly clearing winds fill in behind. Clearing winds occur most often in March, April, and May for a total of about 5–15 times per year. Most SUPers won't appreciate the extreme conditions that come with northwest winds, but for experienced paddlers, these can be fantastic days for shuttled downwind tours.

In general, spring is the windiest time in Southern California, and fall is the least windy. Winter allows for the greatest variance in wind and weather—stormy days are mixed with perfectly glassy days. Summer and early fall have the most consistent weather, but these months are also prone to light-to-moderate afternoon sea breezes.

Several resources are available to aid in determining wind and weather conditions on the water. The **National Data Buoy Center,** a division of the National Oceanic and Atmospheric Administration, produces detailed marine forecasts for Southern California. These reports are updated several times a day and broadcast over a series of weather-radio channels. An online text version of these reports may be found at **tinyurl.com/ndbcforecasts.**

Wind Alert compiles updated wind reports from several weather stations along the Southern California coast. Go to their website, **wind alert.com,** and type in a local zip code to get a detailed map for your area. A subscription is required to access some of the stations, but there are plenty of free wind readings available. Wind Alert is a division of Weather Flow, and their sites **iwindsurf.com** and **ikitesurf.com** also offer wind information. If that isn't enough, all of the sites have free mobile apps so you can get information on the go.

Many shoreline businesses and municipalities have webcams, making it possible to check water conditions before heading to the beach. **Surfline.com** is also a great resource for webcams, offering access to cameras at numerous locations along the Southern California coast. If you intend to launch in the waves, Surfline also provides twice-daily surf reports, updated tide charts, and live wind readings.

Water Temperature

THE CHART ON the following page lists average monthly water temperatures (°F) for various Southern California cities:

City/Beach MONTH	San Clemente	San Diego	Santa Monica	Santa Barbara	Newport Beach	Ventura
Jan	57° F	59° F	57° F	56° F	58° F	55° F
Feb	57° F	61° F	57° F	57° F	60° F	57° F
Mar	58° F	61° F	58° F	57° F	60° F	58° F
Apr	59° F	62° F	59° F	58° F	61° F	59° F
May	61° F	64° F	61° F	60° F	64° F	61° F
Jun 1–15	63° F	65.5° F	63° F	61° F	66° F	62° F
Jun 16–30	63° F	68° F	65° F	62° F	66° F	64° F
Jul	64° F	70° F	66° F	63° F	69° F	64° F
Aug	67° F	72° F	68° F	65° F	69° F	67° F
Sep	66° F	69° F	66° F	64° F	68° F	65° F
Oct 1–15	65° F	69° F	65° F	64° F	68° F	65° F
Oct 16–31	63° F	66° F	63° F	62° F	65° F	62° F
Nov	61° F	65° F	61° F	60° F	64° F	60° F
Dec	58° F	62° F	59° F	57° F	61° F	56° F

Source: *NOAA*

Daily temperatures vary based on local weather conditions, swell events, and upwelling (when cooler deep water is brought to the surface). The mechanics of upwelling are complicated, but the phenomenon often occurs after windy days.

Surf

ALTHOUGH SOUTHERN CALIFORNIA doesn't typically have waves as large as those in Central and Northern California, it does have consistent moderate-sized surf year-round. Typically, south-facing beaches have more surf in the summer, while west-facing beaches tend to pick up winter swells. Parts of Orange County also lie in the shadow of the Channel Islands and therefore aren't exposed to many winter swells.

When you head out in the surf, always check the conditions before venturing into the water. Swells that travel a long distance to

Online Resources for Wave and Swell Information	
magicseaweed.com	stormsurf.com
surfingmagazine/swellwatch	surfline.com

reach our shores often have long intervals between sets. During large surf events, there may also be strong shoreline currents that can make for difficult paddling. If you're uncertain about the conditions, never hesitate to speak with lifeguards or other oceangoers.

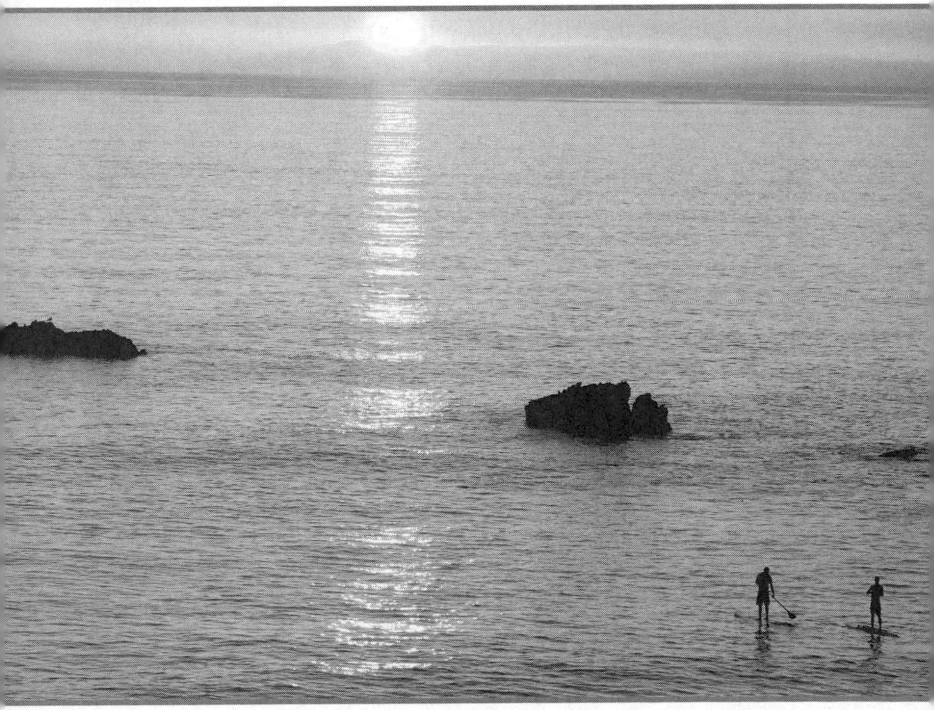

Everything You Ever Wanted to Do on a Stand-Up Board but Were Afraid to Try

THERE'S NOTHING WRONG with simply sitting on the sand and just being near the water. Driving along scenic shorelines and eating dinner at waterside restaurants are nice activities for some folks. For the intrepid, however, it's usually necessary to venture out into the water—to be a boater, a swimmer, a surfer, a diver, an explorer.

If you're one of these types, you already know this: Being on the water is a transformative experience. Whether you're skimming across the surface, diving into the depths, or dropping down the face of a wave, you are somehow defying gravity. You are letting go of the weight of the land and plunging into a separate world—a world that feels different, looks different, and offers myriad unexpected delights.

Of course, there's a downside: It's expensive to buy a boat, it takes time and commitment to learn how to surf, and sometimes jumping into the cold water puts a chill into your body that runs straight down your spine and heads directly into places that we don't even want to talk about. Nevertheless, the hearty and the foolhardy are still out there boating, surfing, and swimming, enduring the costs, the difficulties, and the conditions just so they can be out on the water.

I'm here to tell you that stand-up paddleboards offer one of the easiest and most effective ways to get out on any body of water, and, particularly in Southern California, an ideal way to experience the ocean. No, the boards aren't free, they aren't motorized, and they don't magically appear on the shoreline, but SUP offers a perfect platform to experience a multitude of ocean-related activities: diving, fishing, whale-watching, surfing, exploring, and touring. Whether you want to begin racing or not, the boards offer a fine opportunity to train and improve your physical health. Across the Southland there are SUP yoga classes, SUP fitness classes, and plenty of people just out there paddling with the aim of staying healthy.

What follows is a brief explanation of several SUP-related activities. Whether you are looking to improve your physical fitness, need to relieve some stress, or simply want an opportunity to go out and have fun, there's an SUP activity just for you.

Cruising and Exploring

OBVIOUSLY, SUP IS about getting out on the water. Many enthusiasts are content just doing that—getting away from the beach and feeling the motion of the waves. Cruising around on a stand-up board can be relaxing and liberating. When you stand up, you can peer down into the water, and, on clear days, paddling can be akin to a tour in a glass-bottom boat. Because SUP boards are relatively small (as far as watercraft are concerned), they're capable of navigating through small coves, around rocks, and even between kelp paddies. This is a definite advantage for the ocean explorer, since reefs and rocky shorelines often burst with marine life.

Regardless of the scenery, cruising on an SUP board offers constitutional benefits—an opportunity to skim across the water, to unwind, and to find a bit of needed solace. Not much explanation is necessary: Just go out there and do it.

Fishing

IF FISHING REQUIRES a boat, then an SUP board is essentially a boat that doesn't need a trailer and can be launched almost anywhere. It's a simple solution that has inspired an emerging community of SUP anglers. Not surprisingly, several companies design equipment to suit their needs. SUP fishing accessories include deck-mounted rod holders and board-friendly dry bags that are perfect for transporting equipment out on the water.

Typically, SUP fishermen want a floaty touring-style board to accommodate their gear. For the serious angler, there are specifically designed fishing SUP boards with complete systems to get you and your gear out on the water and catching fish. In lieu of special equipment, some paddlers use low-tech solutions to stow gear. One of the simplest is to put a cooler on board to carry bait, tackle, and, hopefully, fish. This practice may not be recommended for the open ocean (particularly if the cooler can't be secured to the board), but the cooler doubles as a nice seat when you want to take a break.

Diving

NO, YOU CAN'T paddle under water—your SUP board is not a submarine. However, a stand-up board is an effective way to access reefs and kelp beds that are ideal for snorkelers (scuba gear is prohibitively heavy to take on an SUP board). If you're diving off your board into the open ocean, the only caveat is to make sure you don't become separated from the board. The easy solution is to use a leash system—and secure the paddle—and then your board will follow safely behind you. There is so much to explore beneath the surface of the ocean. Having an SUP board gives you much greater mobility, and therefore the ability to take your mask and snorkel to offshore locations that may be out of your swimming range.

Paddling with Whales and Marine Mammals

WHALE-WATCHING HAS INSPIRED a cottage industry in Southern California. On weekends throughout the year, charter boats are packed with camera-toting tourists hoping to spot some of Earth's largest mammals. Although there is never a guarantee of encountering whales on an SUP board, it provides a memorable experience (or experiences) when it happens and is certainly worth trying.

Gray whales follow a fairly dependable pattern, passing through the local waters twice—in the late fall and the early spring—on their round-trip from Alaska to Baja California. The gray-whale population is rather robust these days—around 20,000 individuals—allowing for plenty of sighting opportunities. In the early spring, when accompanied by young calves, the pods often pass quite close to shore.

Blue whales are much more elusive, rarely passing through the near-shore waters. Paddlers who encounter these whales typically have to go 1–2 miles offshore. It's a bit of commitment, but the payoff is great. Blue whales are the largest mammals on the planet. From a distance they can be recognized by their enormous spout, which is easily two times the size of a gray whale's.

Whale-watching boats have the advantage of sonar and spotter planes to seek out pods of marine mammals. Obviously, you don't have these tools on an SUP board, but it never hurts to pay attention to the activity of the whale-watching boats. If you're out paddling and you see crowded slow-moving vessels on the water, this may mean they're tracking whales. Because SUP boards are human-powered, they may travel much closer to the pods than the large motorized crafts. Use this to your advantage—whales are as gentle as they are majestic.

Bottlenose and common dolphins are frequently sighted in the near-shore regions of Southern California. Look for them in the food-rich waters near reefs and kelp beds. Dolphins typically travel in pods, and when food is present, they often feed in a particular area for extended periods of time. Dolphins are also famous acrobats and, on some occasions, can be seen jumping out of the water in graceful arcing motions.

Seals and sea lions also frequent many of our local waters. Colonies of seals can be found in and around harbors and marinas. Sea lions tend to haul out on offshore rocks and sometimes can be found along the beach. When you're out paddling, look for small bubbles rising up in the water—this is often an indication that sea lions are swimming below. (Large bubbles may mean that scuba divers are beneath you.)

Seeing marine mammals in their habitat is a rewarding experience that engenders an appreciation for these beautiful animals and their importance to the planet. Always take care not to harass any animals. Whales and particularly dolphins are very capable swimmers, and it will be difficult, if not impossible, to impede their progress on your paddleboard. Respect sea lion habitats—many sea lions have become accustomed to human interaction, but always stay a healthy distance from their rookeries, so as not to agitate the animals. Finally, note that a lone marine mammal approaching the beach may be sick or injured, so try to give the animal space and, if necessary, call the local fish-and-game office or a marine-mammal rescue center.

Racing

EVERY YEAR IN September, the Southern California SUP community comes together for the **Battle of the Paddle.** It's the biggest SUP event of the year, attracting some of the most prominent names in the sport. Competitors come from across the Southland, as well as from Hawaii, Canada, and Europe. The exciting series of races requires paddlers to navigate through the surf, make buoy turns, and even run across the sand.

In 2014, the event was held at Salt Creek Beach in Dana Point. A large south swell was pumping, and the conditions made for a race that was equal parts chaotic and exciting. A thousand-plus spectators lined the beach, cheering on the competitors and marveling at the spectacle. Aside from a bit of jousting in the men's final, there was amazing camaraderie among the paddlers. Everyone out there on a board seemed to be having the time of their lives. If ever there was a scene that would inspire one to take up SUP racing, this was it.

Although it has expanded in recent years, the racing component of stand-up paddling nearly dates back to the introduction of the sport to Southern California. More than any other aspect of SUP-ing, racing has promoted a community of paddlers. Paddling competitions bring people together to test their abilities and to celebrate the virtues of the sport. For paddlers of all ages and abilities, racing is a great motivational tool—to paddle, to train, and to stay fit.

If you're excited about the sport and looking to find other like-minded individuals, try signing up for one of the numerous SUP competitions. Because of the favorable weather in Southern California, SUP events go on nearly year-round. You don't need to own a specialized race board—most competitions have an all-encompassing surfboard class designed for beginning paddlers with less-performance-oriented boards. There are races in flat-water locales such as Mission Bay, races that begin in marinas and venture out into the ocean, and races such as the Battle of the Paddle that run courses through the surf. There really is something for everyone: distance races, ultradistance races, downwind races, and even an obstacle race. The common element in every competition is that people get together and partake in one of their favorite activities.

Check out Appendix 3 (page 203) for a month-by-month listing of SUP racing events. For additional listings, see **supracer.com** or **paddleguru.com.**

SUP Yoga

YOGA HAS SUCCEEDED as a land-based practice for roughly 5,000 years. So, to the casual observer, it might seem unnecessary to take this time-honored discipline and move it out onto the water. However, performing yoga poses on paddleboards can be an engaging experience. Obviously SUP yoga will never usurp mat-based yoga, but the practice on water offers several amazing benefits.

First of all, SUP yoga is a challenging and beneficial workout. Performing poses on the water requires additional balance, strength, and concentration. Because the board is constantly moving, staying in balance requires significant muscle energy. As you move through poses on the board, your entire midsection must work hard to keep you level on the water. There is no discounting the physical benefits of traditional yoga, but practicing SUP yoga will force you to effectively work your core muscle group and to strengthen and develop fast-twitch muscles.

Being on the water also offers a great deal of serenity. Not only are you out in nature, but you are floating. The motion of the water becomes an added benefit to the experience. Certainly there is a slight fear factor in balancing on an unstable board. But it's only water—you aren't balancing over hot lava—and getting wet may just be part of the process.

If you already do traditional yoga, practicing poses on an SUP board will force you to refine your technique. Asanas (yoga poses) that you may have taken for granted will take on new dimensions on the water. Rebooting your practice anew may seem intimidating, but it can also be instructive—to let go of your preconceived notions and adopt a beginner's mind-set is a powerful learning tool.

In general, SUP yoga offers many of the same advantages of regular stand-up paddling—it's an opportunity to get away, to get out on the water, to exercise, and to have fun.

Surfing

MAYBE THE MOST dynamic and challenging offshoot of SUP, stand-up surfing has undergone an amazing evolution in the last several years. Although it may seem easy, there is definitely a learning curve for surfing on a stand-up board. There are also safety concerns. Before taking your SUP board into the surf, you need to understand the rules of the game—essentially how to safely coexist with other surfers and stand-up surfers in the water. This may require general wave knowledge, an understanding of surf etiquette, and even a bit of local knowledge. See page 147 for an introduction to stand-up-surfing techniques, and see "A SoCal SUS Sampler" (page 159) for descriptions of various Southern California surf breaks.

Paddling the Southland

THE FOLLOWING CHAPTERS detail some of the many beaches, harbors, and waterways to SUP in Southern California. The locations run from north to south, beginning with San Diego Harbor (**Coronado Tidelands Park**) and stretching all the way to northern Santa Barbara County (**Refugio State Beach**). For each area, I've listed destinations that are suitable for all types of users.

Of course, you may find other spots on your own, but think of the ones that follow as a jumping-off point—an invitation to go out and paddle, to get outdoors, and to explore our magnificent coast.

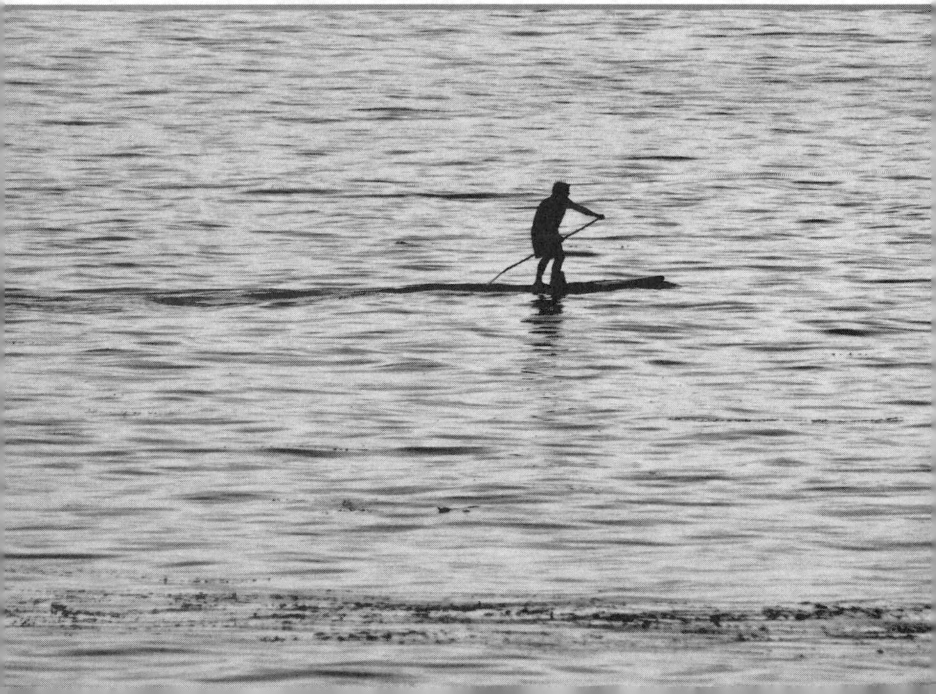

San Diego County

The public dock for launching kayaks and paddleboards in Oceanside Harbor (see page 63)

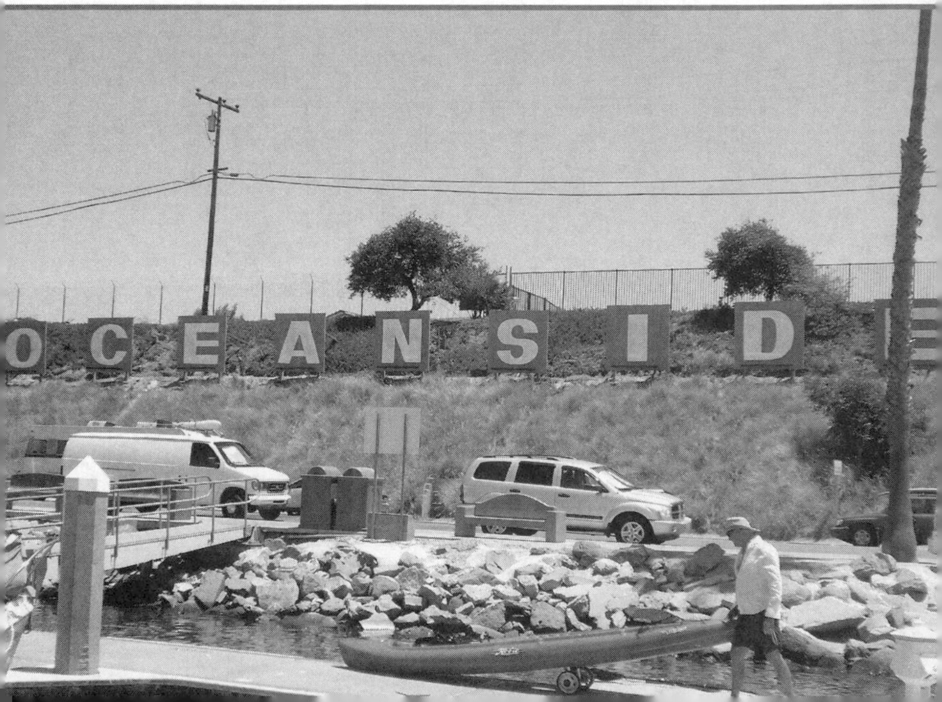

Coronado Tidelands Park

Coronado

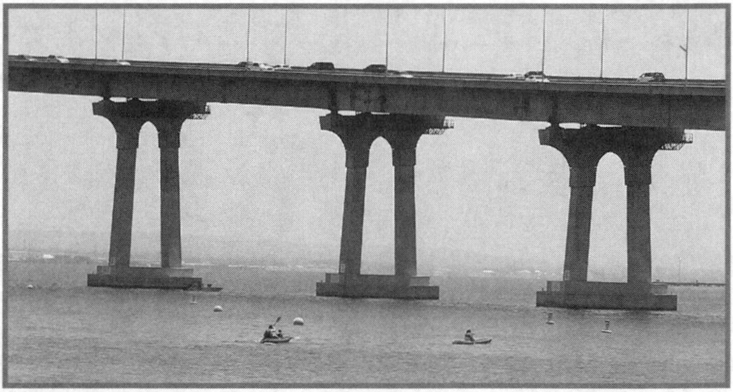

The Coronado Bridge

OVERVIEW It's easy to feel small when paddling in San Diego Harbor. The city skyline towers to the east, impossibly large naval ships sit in wait at Indian Point, and the Coronado Bridge spans high above the water.

WHERE TO PADDLE When launching at Coronado Tidelands Park, paddlers set out in the shadow of the bridge—the beach is a mere few hundred feet from the most westward footings—and it's hard to ignore the constant hum of vehicles passing back and forth above the water. Of course, if the sound is bothersome, it's only a short paddle to quieter waters.

The sandy beach at the park, with its calm protected shore, is fairly ideal for launching paddleboards. There is also nearby parking and a nice grassy area with shade and restrooms. The conditions on the water are definitely beginner-friendly, but not as easy as, say, Mission Bay (see page 49). Even though San Diego Harbor is protected, its vast size makes it inclined to wind and chop. It's also possible that the size and scale of the waterway may intimidate some who are new to the sport—fear not, though, as long as you stay reasonably close to shore. For those wanting to venture far offshore, even experienced paddlers should be cautious when heading into the shipping channel. Big ships move fast and they're, well, big.

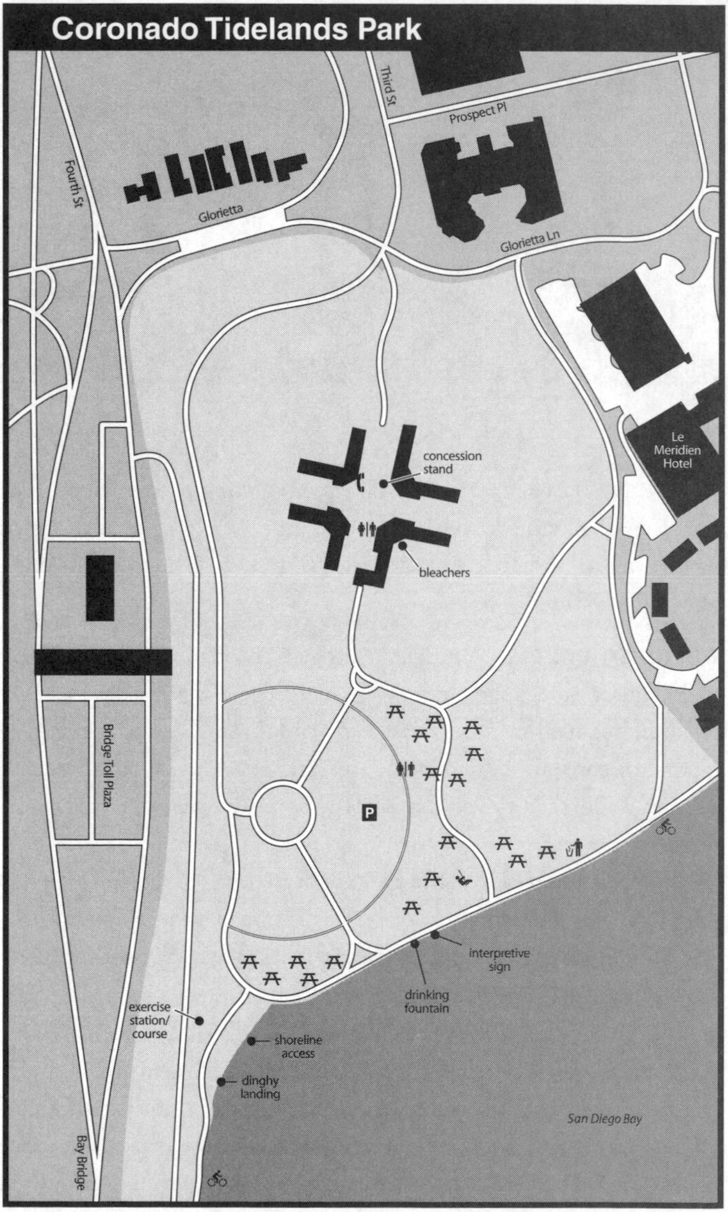
Coronado Tidelands Park
Third St
Prospect Pl
Fourth St
Glorietta
Glorietta Ln
Le
Meridien
Hotel
concession
stand
bleachers
Bridge Toll Plaza
P
interpretive
sign
drinking
fountain
exercise
station/
course
shoreline
access
dinghy
landing
San Diego Bay
Bay Bridge

Most beginners will probably prefer paddling south and west from the Tidelands beach, under the bridge, and into the relatively calm waters of **Glorietta Bay.** Even on a moderately breezy day, after passing under the bridge and turning westward, I found calm conditions in the inlet of the bay. Most of the other paddlers I saw were also in this area—many of them renting boards at the Coronado Boathouse at the west end of the inlet. The western shoreline of the bay follows the boundary of a golf course. Beyond the sights of the bridge and the naval yard, it isn't the most scenic place to paddle, but it is easy and fairly free of boat traffic.

Paddling to the north from the beach (toward Point Loma) may require more effort depending on conditions, but those heading toward the upper section of the island will be rewarded with nice views of the San Diego skyline. Boat enthusiasts also may enjoy checking out some of the local marine traffic. One Friday afternoon, I watched the *Stars and Stripes,* defender of the 1995 America's Cup, tack back and forth just west of the bridge. Indeed, this is a very active waterway. Sharing the water with commercial traffic, naval traffic, and pleasure boats may cause paddlers to feel small but certainly not bored.

DIRECTIONS AND PARKING From I-5 South, take CA 75 South over the expansive bridge to the island of Coronado. Once you're on the island, head through the empty tollbooths—there is no longer a toll—and then take the first right onto Glorietta Boulevard. Once on Glorietta, take the first right on Mullinex Drive. This will take you into the park. Stay to the right and park near the skate park. The sandy beach will be directly in front of you, in the direction of the bridge.

Note: When driving in Coronado, pay close attention to speed limits, stop signs, and parking restrictions. The local police here are known for their citation-writing skills. Parking is free and generally available. There are also restrooms, picnic tables, and a grassy area with plenty of shade.

CONDITIONS AND HAZARDS The launch is sandy and easy to manage. The main channel of the harbor can get a bit choppy, but nearby Glorietta Bay has plenty of smooth water. Most paddlers will want to stay close to shore, avoiding the large ships in the main channel.

RENTALS At this writing, there is no board-rental agency at Coronado Tidelands Park, but the **Coronado Club Room and Boathouse,** on nearby Glorietta Bay (1985 Strand Way; 619-522-2655, **tinyurl.com/ccrboathouse**), has SUP boards for rent ($30 for 2 hours or $75 for an entire day).

LOCAL BURRITO I used to travel to Baja California quite frequently. Near the end of every trip, after arriving in San Diego, I would stop at **El Indio** (3695 India St.; 619-299-0333, **elindiosandiego.com**). This was the Mexican food I would eat after leaving Mexico. A tortilla factory and restaurant, El Indio is a San Diego institution, having served customers since 1940. They're known for their taquitos as well as their handmade tortilla chips, which are always thick and always fresh. I still recommend ordering a burrito, however. (I am committed to the cause.) Choose from around a dozen varieties, including carnitas, carne asada, grilled chicken, and fish.

The San Diego skyline as viewed from the park

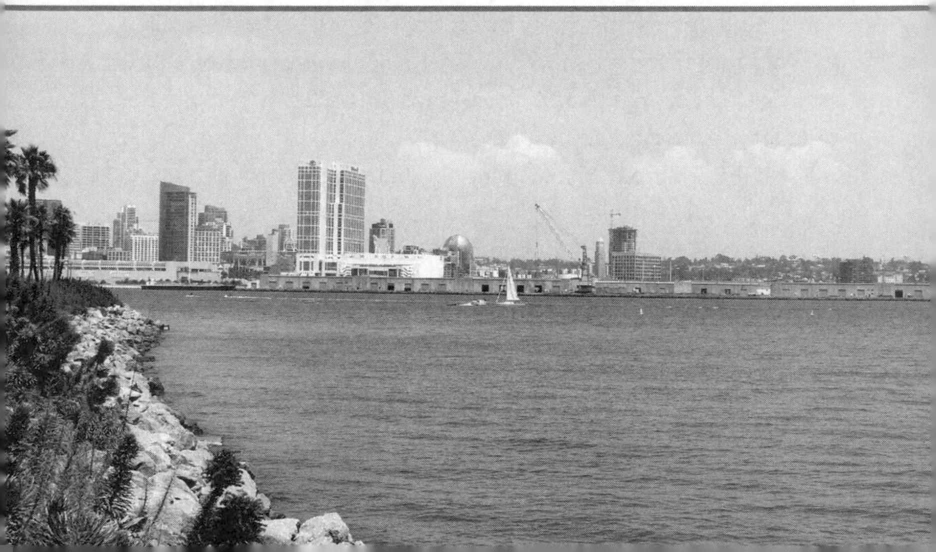

Mission Bay San Diego

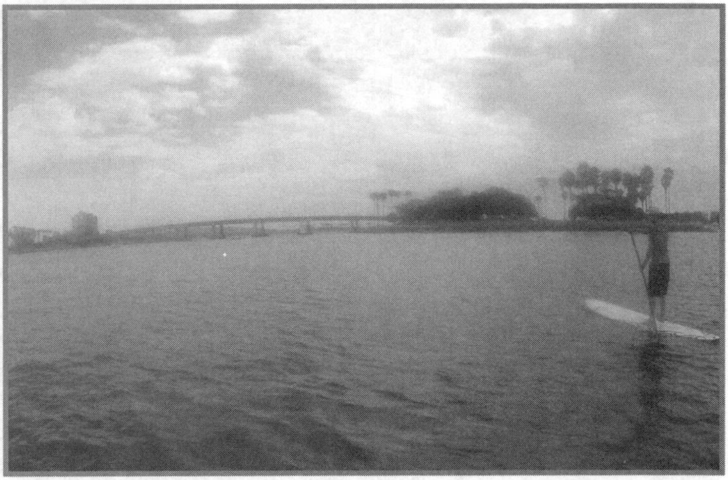

Paddling near Vacation Island in Mission Bay

OVERVIEW The first thing to know about Mission Bay is that it is huge. With 4,200 acres of water, islands, and peninsulas and more than 27 miles of shoreline, Mission Bay is the largest aquatic park in the country. Despite its immense size, the waterway is easily navigated.

WHERE TO PADDLE For stand-up paddling, it's best to remain in **Sail Bay,** accessible from Mission Bay Drive in Pacific Beach. Fiesta Bay, which makes up most of the eastern portion of the aquatic park, is a haven for water-skiers, Jet-Skiers, and powerboat users. Sail Bay has much more restrictive speed limits, with only the occasional catamaran topping the 5-miles-per-hour threshold.

Although there is plenty of beach space along the western edge of Sail Bay, **Santa Clara Point** remains the primary hub for SUP activity. The point is home to Mission Bay Sportcenter and Mission Bay Aquatic Center. Both of these outfitters offer SUP rentals, as well as lessons and camps for kids. (They also support a myriad of other water sports—from sailing to surf lessons to jet pack rentals.) For paddlers with their own equipment, Santa Clara Point offers easy beach access, with an adequate stretch of sandy shoreline and plenty of lawn space

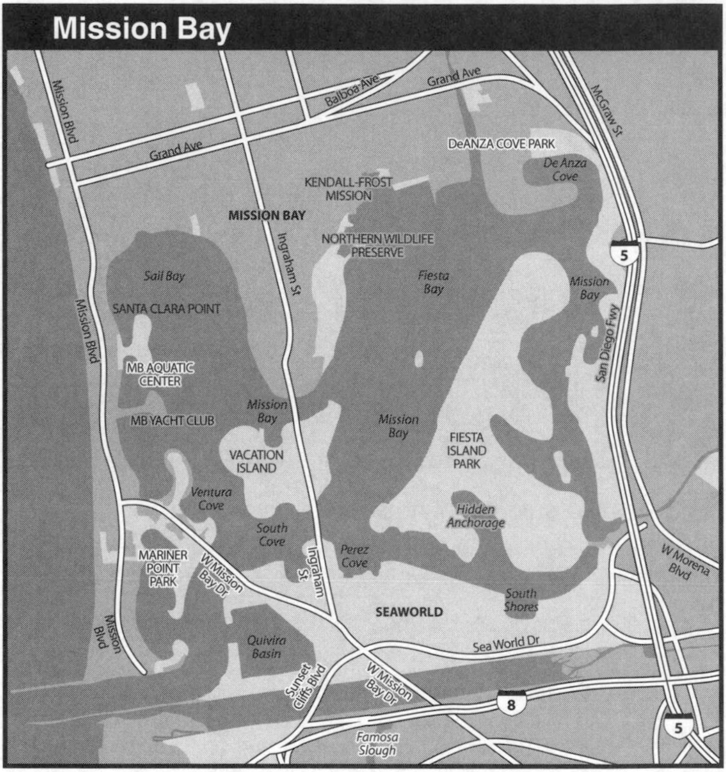

to leave boards, beach gear, or family members. Parking is available in lots near the Sportcenter and the Aquatic Center, but the spaces will fill up on busy summer weekends (On a Friday afternoon in July, I needed to muster a bit of patience before I secured a spot.)

The paddling experience in Mission Bay is neither challenging nor overly stimulating, but it is pleasant—a perfect place for beginners, families, SUP yoga enthusiasts, and just about anyone who wants to train on open stretches of flat water. It's hard to overestimate the opportunities for family recreation in Mission Bay. At both the Aquatic Center and the Sportcenter, there are child camps galore. Expect to see groups of kids paddling, surfing (it's a short walk to the ocean), swimming, and running about. For families with their own stand-up boards, Santa Clara Point is a perfect place to picnic, paddle, and maybe throw a Frisbee.

Most of Sail Bay lies to the south of Santa Clara Point. Heading in that direction, paddlers will soon cross the shores of the **Mission Bay Yacht Club.** Here, if there is an ounce of wind to be had, expect to encounter a bevy of small sailboats, part of the club's extensive sailing school. A Friday afternoon found a fleet of young Sabot sailors, tipping their way through a few jibes. Sail Bay is appropriately named and, beyond the shores of the yacht club, there are plenty of larger sailboats on the water, including a fair concentration of catamarans. Fortunately, even though the area is popular with sailboats, the wind in Mission Bay tends to be light, steady, and typically cross-shore. Even when sailors are out on the water, conditions can be fine for paddling.

Farther south one finds **Vacation Island** (to the east), home to Paradise Isle, a large resort with swimming pools and waterfalls that seems to cater to SeaWorld visitors. The eastern portion of Vacation Island also includes a city park with lawns and picnic benches overlooking the water. This public portion of the island may be accessed from Ingraham Street (although launching a paddleboard here means heading out among the powerboats in Fiesta Bay). The two prominent landmarks beyond Vacation Island include the aforementioned **SeaWorld** and **Fiesta Island.** The theme park, famous for its captive orcas and dolphins, isn't visible from the water, but paddlers should recognize the observation spire peaking above the trees in the distance. Fiesta Island, visible just to the east of Vacation Island, is a large, sandy expanse that plays host to San Diego's annual Over the Line Tournament. The event, which is more about bawdy behavior and beer than any sort of athletics—is a bit of an onus for the city. Every year they try to curtail the bad behavior, and every year people come hoping for more.

After about a mile, paddlers will reach the **Mission Street Bridge.** Ahead is the entrance channel that leads to the breakwater and the Pacific Ocean (still another mile away). The channel isn't particularly scenic but will have a greater concentration of boat traffic—fishing charters, pleasure boats, and (when they are practicing) teams of outrigger canoes. Overall, Mission Bay has enough space for paddlers who want to race and train, but it is also safe and sane for boarders of all ages and ability levels. This isn't La Jolla—don't expect to be blown away by the scenery. Paddlers who come here should do so because they want things to be easy and relaxing.

DIRECTIONS AND PARKING From I-5 South, exit at Mission Bay Drive and turn right on Garnet Avenue. Follow Garnet as it becomes Balboa Avenue and then merges onto Grand Avenue. At 2.2 miles from the freeway, turn left onto Mission Boulevard. After another 0.9 mile, turn left at Santa Clara Place. Mission Bay Aquatic Center will be directly on the right. To get to the Mission Bay Sportcenter, take the first left and head along the water to the parking lot. Parking is free but will be in short supply on busy days.

CONDITIONS AND HAZARDS Relaxing and family-friendly, Mission Bay should appeal to those who want things to be simple and easy. You may find quite a few boats on the water in Sail Bay, but there's plenty of space to navigate around them. Even most windy days aren't *that* windy, but afternoon sea breezes might produce a bit of bump on the water.

Short of an orca escaping from SeaWorld (one can hope), the waters seem safe. During large winter swells, waves will form inside the harbor mouth; this is a long way from the launch at Santa Clara Point, however. Years ago the local outrigger crews would, on occasion, ride these waves into the harbor. That was until one crew crashed their outrigger into the jetty. The whole event was captured by a local news station. Some of the paddlers were able to scramble to safety, and others were picked out of the water by the Harbor Patrol. Thankfully, the only injuries were to the outrigger; since then, however, the outrigger clubs are banned from riding waves inside the Mission Bay jetty. No word on whether anyone in the local SUP community has tried the same.

RENTALS **Mission Bay Aquatic Center** (1001 Santa Clara Place; 858-488-1000, **mbaquaticcenter.com**) offers SUP skills courses as well as

SUP yoga and fitness classes. Board rentals run $26 for 2½ hours; package deals and discounts for UCSD and SDSU students are also available.

Mission Bay Sportcenter (1010 Santa Clara Place; 858-488-1004, **missionbaysportcenter.com**) offers rentals for $15 per hour or $60 per day. They also conduct SUP yoga classes in the morning and SUP tours at night (with lights).

LOCAL BURRITO Forget that the place has *taco* in its name: **Taco Surf Taco Shop** (4657 Mission Blvd.; 858-272-3877, **tacosurftacoshop.com**) was noted on Fox News as making one of the best burritos in America. That may be an overstatement, but it's still a great place to eat (*USA Today* also gave it accolades). The owner, who still works the counter, is an old surfer who affectionately refers to all his customers as "bud" or "dear." Pictures of him surfing the local break line the wall, and his amazing collection of surfboards covers the ceiling. (If this weren't an eatery, it could be a surfboard museum. Seriously.) Try the California burrito, stuffed with carnitas, hash browns, sour cream, and guacamole.

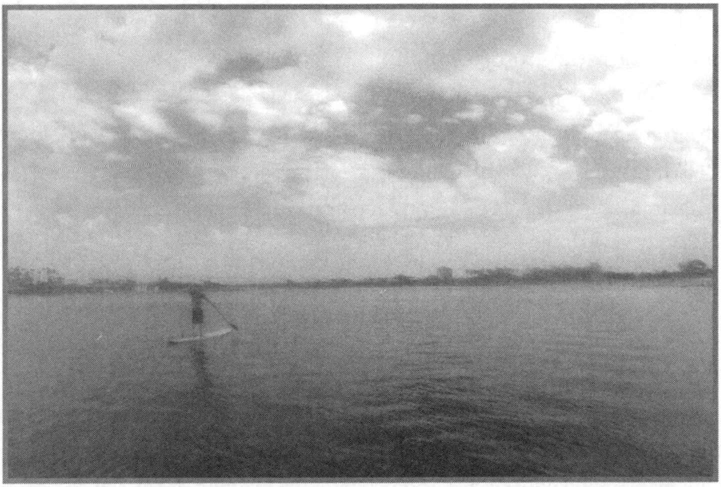

Calm waters in the Sail Bay portion of the bay

LA JOLLA **San Diego**

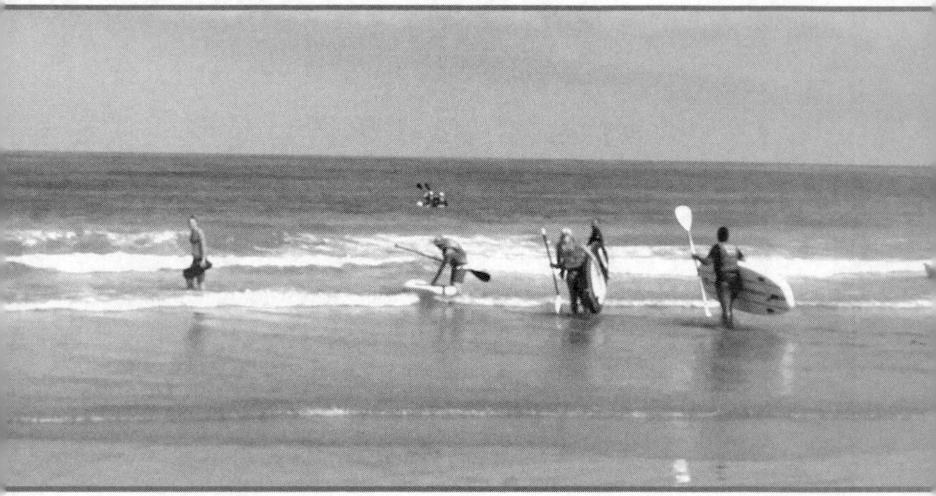

Paddlers entering the water at the La Jolla boat launch

OVERVIEW Not far from downtown San Diego is a waterfront with postcard-perfect cliffs, where sea lions sun themselves amid scenic sea caves and pristine blue water. The waterfront also has a small, protected cove—a perfect location for swimming and snorkeling. All this exists at La Jolla, a place that possesses all the elements for an ideal beach-vacation destination. Of course, everyone knows this, and when the weather is warm, the beaches at La Jolla swarm with tourists. Potential visitors, be forewarned: There will be crowds, there will be traffic, and while there is a decent amount of free parking in the area, there's not enough to accommodate everyone.

WHERE TO PADDLE Caveat aside, La Jolla is a great place to visit and to paddle. The launch at La Jolla Shores provides access to the **La Jolla Ecological Reserve**—6,000 acres of sandy flats, reefs, kelp forest, and glorious underwater habitat. And that's just what lies below the surface. Above is one of the most scenic stretches of coastline in Southern California. Of course, this isn't lost on the local paddling outfitters, who every day send off a virtual armada of tourists, mostly in kayaks, from the boat ramp just south of Kellogg Park.

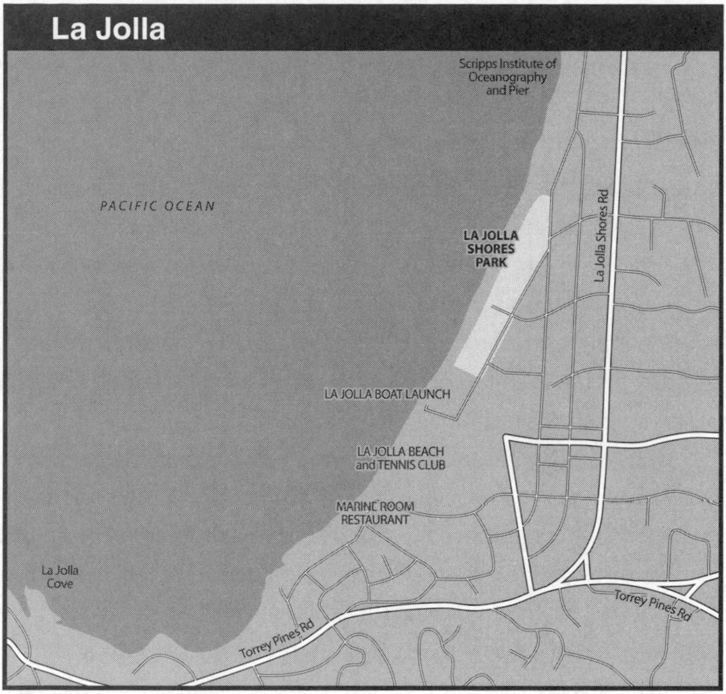

The typical paddle tour puts in at the boat ramp, then heads up to the cliffs and caves that bend around the north side of **La Jolla Cove.** On two separate weekday mornings in July, some 100 kayaks were plying the waters along this stretch, all color-coordinated in the matching reds, blues, and yellows of their tour companies. (The kayak-tour operators also offer SUP, but it seems the majority of their clients take the seated option.)

The crowds on the water shouldn't make you skittish, though; it's fairly easy to find space on the water away from the kayak packs—the tour groups tend to stay together, close to their narrating guides. Of course, the general beach crowd will add a challenge to getting to the water. So my advice is: If you are going in the summer (or even a sunny weekend in the off-season), try to get out early; avoid summer weekends if at all possible; and if you do get caught in the scramble of traffic and limited parking, make the best of it. You can always drop your boards at the boat launch while you search for parking. If that doesn't work, you might try to find parking at the alternate launching area near The Marine Room (see below).

LAUNCHING The beach in front of Kellogg Park is typically packed with swimmers and bathers, so don't try to launch there. Instead, take your boards to the boat launch at the end of **Avenida de la Playa.** There is short-term (15-minute) parking available on the street for those loading and unloading. It's also legal to drive out onto the sand, but this option is generally intended for boat owners and not really necessary for those hauling SUP boards.

The kayak companies stage directly adjacent to the launch, so there may be several tour groups heading out through the surf when you put in the water. If it's too crowded, try to find some open beach just south of the boat launch. (This should be pretty apparent when you're at the launch.) As far as getting through the surf, the gentle, sloping beach makes for slow-rolling (read: friendly) surf, so getting outside should be easy on most days. The sandy beach is perfect for tender feet, but the area is also prone to stingrays. Be sure to shuffle your feet when entering and exiting the water. Once you are outside the break, try to respect the swim boundaries of the **La Jolla Beach & Tennis Club.**

If the boat launch seems too crowded or parking is just impossible, a second option is to launch near **The Marine Room** restaurant, on the south side of the Beach & Tennis Club. Limited free street parking is available nearby on Spindrift Drive and on Roseland Street; once parked, head down the narrow beach access that abuts the south side of the restaurant. The launch here is not terribly different from the aforementioned boat launch, but you may find surfers in the water. It's somewhat of a beginner break, and it may also be frequented by families staying at the club, so respect their space, trying to put in and paddle away from the surfing lineup. This may mean heading out just south of the beach access. There are some offshore reefs here, and the area is popular with stand-up surfers (see the section on La Jolla

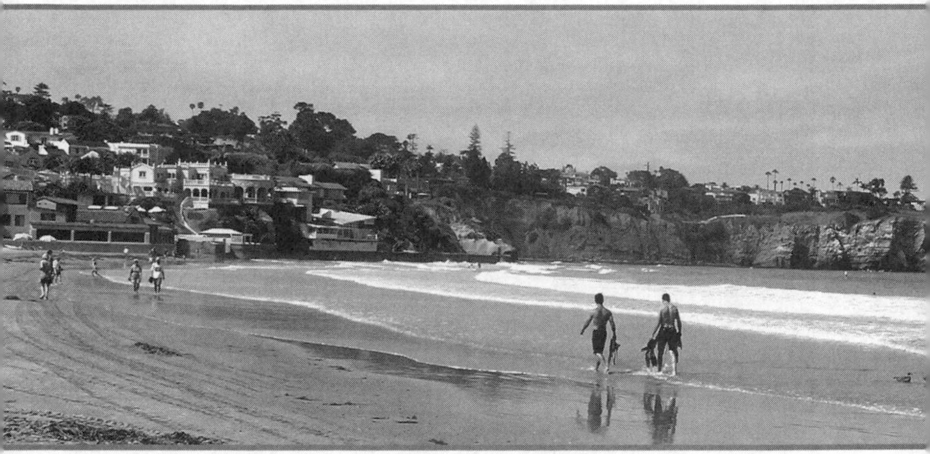

The beach in front of the La Jolla Beach and Tennis Club. La Jolla Cove is in the distance.

Shores in "A SoCal SUS Sampler," page 163), but the conditions are generally friendly for those who simply want to push through the surf and tour the outer waters of the ecological park.

From either of the launches, the paddle toward the caves and La Jolla Cove takes about 20–30 minutes. The caves are magnificent and larger than you might expect. The largest inlet is supposedly navigable at high tide (it wasn't either of the times I was there).

Beyond the cliffs are the sea lions and the famous little cove at La Jolla. There will be plenty of snorkelers inside the cove, so avoid paddling in close. (If you do, expect to get an earful from the lifeguards.) For those wanting to paddle and snorkel, take advantage of your board and start your dive near one of the offshore kelp beds. (Be sure to use a leash when doing this—you want to remain with your board in the open ocean.) Also, a small inlet just below the main cove (near the sea lion area) typically has just a few snorkelers, so this might be a paddling and diving option as well.

DIRECTIONS AND PARKING *To the boat launch at 2000 Avenida de la Playa:* Exit I-5 at La Jolla Village Drive. Head west on La Jolla

Village for 0.7 mile, and then turn left on Torrey Pines Road. Continue for 2 miles. Turn right onto Camino de la Plata. After 0.3 mile, veer left onto Avenida de la Playa. The road ends at the sand. There is 15-minute parking on both sides of the street on the block west of Camino Del Oro. To get to the parking lot at La Jolla Shores Park, head north on Camino Del Oro for 0.2 mile before turning left into the parking lot entrance. Parking is free, but the lot may be crowded.

To the beach access near The Marine Room: Follow the above directions to Torrey Pines Road. After 2.2 miles, turn right onto Little Street. Follow Little Street as it veers left, then take the first right onto St. Louis Terrace. After 0.1 mile, turn right on Spindrift Drive and look for parking. The Marine Room (2000 Spindrift Drive) will be straight ahead on the left. The beach access is on the south side of the restaurant.

CONDITIONS AND HAZARDS Open-ocean conditions are the norm, but the waves are typically gentle. The cliffs provide a buffer against south winds. Expect to see crowds of kayaks on the water and a high concentration of snorkelers in La Jolla Cove.

Watch out for stingrays when launching, and avoid aggravated drivers when parking. Just north of the cliffs are some offshore reefs that can produce rolling—and occasionally breaking—swells. When launching near The Marine Room, try to steer clear of any packs of surfers. (It shouldn't be too difficult, but it is a useful consideration.)

RENTALS AND LESSONS Izzy Tihanyi, co-owner of **Surf Diva Surf Shop,** is an avid practitioner of stand-up paddling and an enthusiastic proponent of paddling in La Jolla. (It's hard to overestimate her love of the sport. If you don't believe me, just ask her.) Her shop, just two short blocks from the boat launch, offers board rentals, basic SUP lessons, and stand-up-surfing lessons. Lessons tend to be private or in small groups. The rental fleet covers a wide range of board shapes and styles. Surf Diva also carries its own line of boards. (2160 Avenida de la Playa; 858-454-8273, **surfdiva.com.**)

Agua Hedionda Carlsbad

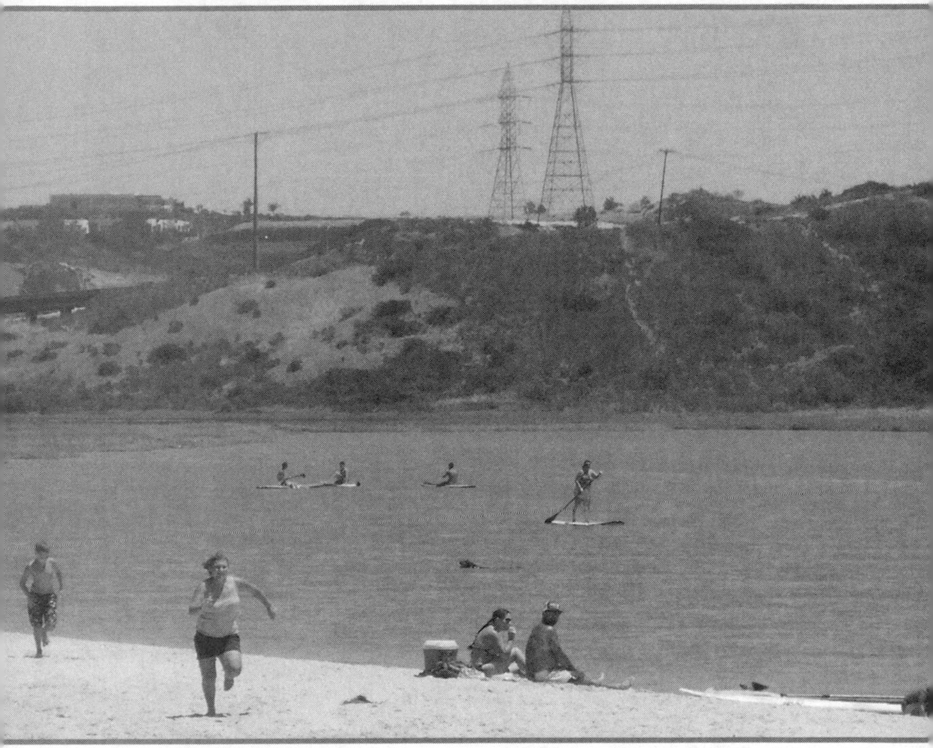

The prime launching spot and dog-friendly beach at Bayshore Drive

OVERVIEW *Agua hedionda* means "stinking water" in Spanish, but Agua Hedionda Lagoon hasn't been smelly in decades. In 1954, the upper waterway was dredged and two stone jetties were constructed to ensure proper drainage to the ocean. This is necessary since, apart from recreational use, the lagoon is home to a thriving aquaculture business. Carlsbad Aquafarm raises abalone, clams, mussels, oysters, and edible seaweeds in the western portion of the lagoon.

The lagoon is also an ecological preserve that provides refuge to more than 200 types of migratory birds. It's a serene, fairly uncrowded waterway, a perfect paddling spot for those not wanting to deal with crowds or challenging conditions.

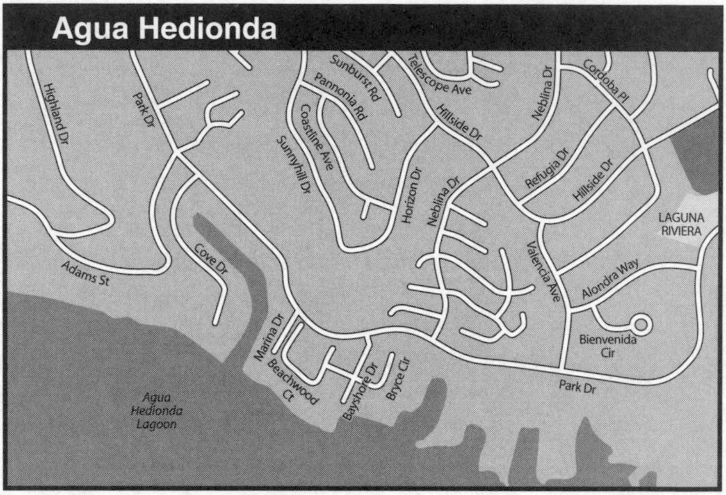

WHERE TO PADDLE The larger section of the lagoon, which lies to the east of Interstate 5, is a nature preserve with separate sections carved out for boating and paddling (boats and Jet-Skis are restricted to the area closest to I-5). Paddlers have been allotted space farther inland, in the shallower, calmer, and, frankly, more scenic section of the lagoon. Paddlers with their own boards may access the lagoon at **Bayshore Drive.** Just park in the cul-de-sac and follow a short pathway that leads to the sandy beach. A sign directs users to launch within 35 feet of the walkway—curious, as there are several hundred feet of beach frontage. On the day I was there, paddlers were heading out along the entire stretch of sand, so perhaps the sign is only appropriate when sand is lacking. Either way, Agua Hedionda Lagoon is an appropriate place for beginning paddlers, with calm waters and an easy and accessible launch.

The waterway has ample space to paddle, but it's still small enough that one would never get lost or paddle too far and become tired. Adults with children will appreciate the sandy beach and the good sight lines between the shore and the water. The beach at Bayshore Drive is also dog-friendly, but dogs must be leashed.

For paddlers seeking rentals, instruction, fitness classes, and yoga classes, the **Carlsbad Paddle Club** is the place. About 1 mile west of the Bayshore Drive launch, the paddle club is currently leased by the **Floating Yogis** and local SUP sensations **2 Stand Up Guys** (see Rentals and Lessons below).

DIRECTIONS AND PARKING To reach Bayshore Drive, exit I-5 at Tamarack Avenue and head east. After 0.4 mile, turn right onto Highland Drive and continue onto Hillside Drive. Take the first right onto Park Drive and continue 0.6 mile to Bayshore Drive. Turn right and park as close to the lagoon as possible. See **tinyurl.com/aguahedionda** for a map of the area.

The 2 Stand Up Guys and the Floating Yogis are located at 4509 Adams St. Exit I-5 at Tamarack, then take the first right at Adams Street. Continue 0.8 mile to the signed driveway for the Carlsbad Paddling Club. Head down the narrow drive about 200 feet to the small parking lot.

RENTALS AND LESSONS Marci and Sarah, the **Floating Yogis,** offer various types of paddleboard yoga classes—kids, adults, teacher training—on the lagoon. Paddles and boards are included. Call 760-525-8625 or check their website, **floatingyogis.com,** for details.

The **2 Stand Up Guys** are Matt Poth and Ryan Judson. They're not only SUP enthusiasts but also generous and knowledgeable instructors. Their Carlsbad operation includes children's camps and a school-based physical education program known as ISPE (Independent Stand-Up Paddling Physical Education). They're also starting an SUP instructor-training program and offer private and group instruction in various other San Diego locations. Paddles and boards are included. Their website, **2standupguys.com** (phone: 347-489-3926), provides information on their business as well as fun video tutorials for stand-up surfers. It's worth checking out.

HAZARDS None, really. Paddle too far west and you may encounter boats and Jet-Skis, but the various usage areas are well signed and far apart.

LOCAL BURRITO Chefs always insist that "fat is flavor." For Mexican food, the saying might be "lard is luscious." The chile relleno burrito at **Armando's Mexican Food** is filled with creamy *manteca*-intensive refried beans and wrapped in a rich (you guessed it—more lard) flour tortilla. It's a mouthful of comfort and spice—probably about 1,000 calories worth—for only $4. Armando's won't wow you with atmosphere, but for value and tasty food, it's hard to beat. (1426 Mission Ave., Oceanside; 760-967-9340.)

Access to the beach and the lagoon at Bayshore Drive

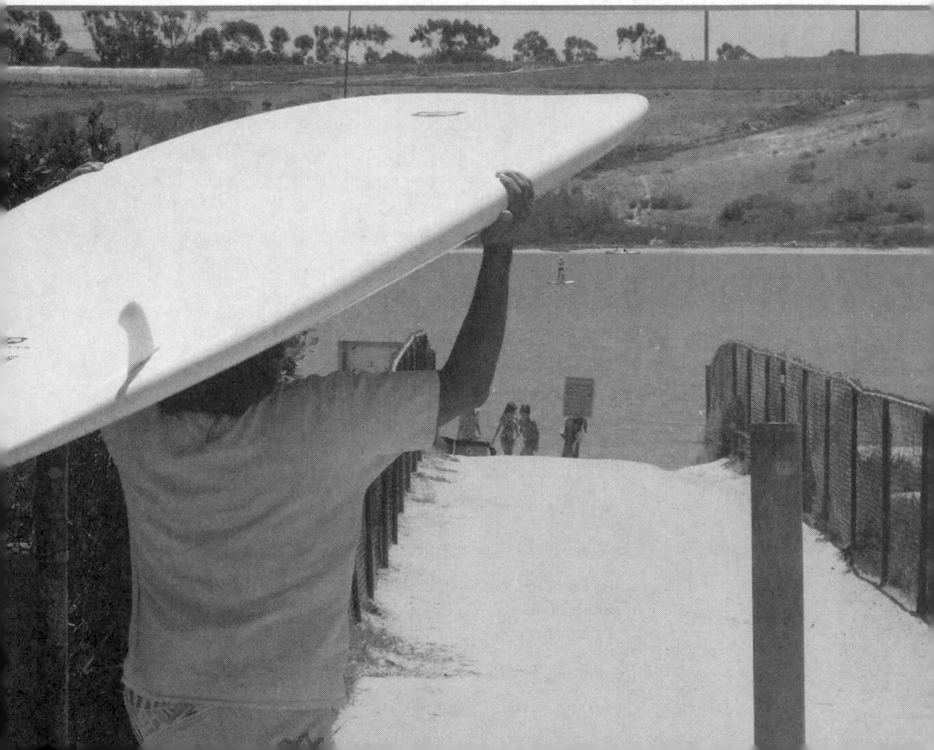

Oceanside Harbor

Oceanside

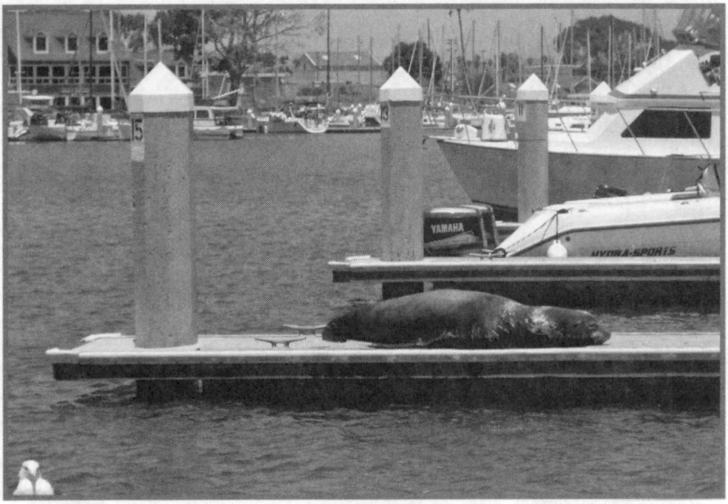

A lazy sea lion suns itself near the launching area.

OVERVIEW Harbors and marinas all look similar from a distance: plenty of boats, a few piers, a jetty, and at least one nautically themed restaurant selling fish and chips. That doesn't mean they're all the same, though. Each harbor has its own personality, and Oceanside Harbor might draw comparisons to a sleepy retirement park in central Florida. The pace is relaxed. On warm summer days, expect to see a mature set of kayakers on the water and perhaps a few children fishing from the dock with their grandparents. This is a place where time moves slowly amid the sunshine and blue water—at least until happy hour starts at the local Jolly Roger restaurant.

WHERE TO PADDLE The shore of the harbor is rocky, but there is a launching pier for paddleboards (and kayaks). Just follow North Harbor Drive past the fishing pier and look for the public launch, directly below the blue OCEANSIDE sign. There is street parking nearby and a public restroom about 100 feet south of the launch.

As per a sign on the dock, all paddlers must wear personal flotation devices while out in the harbor. (I'm not sure if the rule is enforced, but most everyone on the water seems to comply. On a

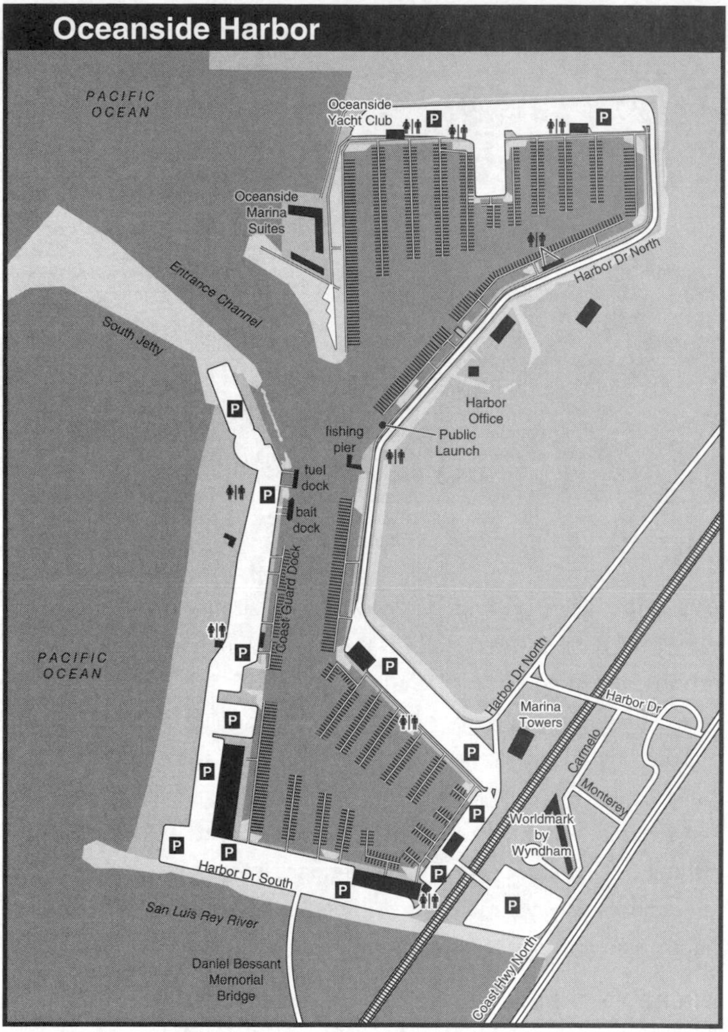

weekday afternoon, most of the SUP boards on the water were from rental companies.) The sign also instructs paddlers to launch quickly and not to block access to the water, but there is no sense of rush at the dock. When I was there, adults and children went out and came in at a leisurely pace. The only ruckus was caused by a barking sea lion, who merely wanted a chance to lie in the sun. (He found some empty dock space nearby.)

The launch and conditions are perfectly easy and friendly for beginners. Most paddlers either tour through the rows of slip spaces, or head out toward the harbor mouth. The layout of the harbor is fairly basic and therefore easy to navigate. The only hazard might be a few speeding Jet-Skis. When heading toward the harbor mouth, I would suggest staying to the north side of the channel and inside of the no-wake zone (watch for signs and buoys). Otherwise, enjoy the calm conditions and laid-back atmosphere. And if it gets too windy in the afternoon, just remember that the Jolly Roger happy hour begins at 3 o'clock.

DIRECTIONS AND PARKING Exit I-5 at Oceanside Harbor Drive and head west. At the first intersection, head left—don't go into Camp Pendleton—and down the hill, then veer right onto North Harbor Drive. Follow this road for about a mile. The public dock is directly below the OCEANSIDE sign. Free street parking is available. See **tinyurl.com/oceansideharbor** for a map of the area.

CONDITIONS AND HAZARDS Calm waters and plenty of space prevail. It's perfect for the whole family. PFDs are required. Big sea lions mostly want to be left alone. Jet-Skis should definitely be left alone.

RENTALS **Boat Rentals of America** (256 Harbor Drive S.; 760-722-0028, **boats4rent.com/oceanside**) rents wide, stable, beginner-friendly paddleboards for $25 per hour ($40 for 2 hours). PFDs are provided. The rental agency is at the other end of the harbor from the public launch; the upside is that it has its own convenient launch area.

LOCAL BURRITO **Armando's Mexican Food** (1426 Mission Ave.; 760-967-9340): See page 62 for details.

Orange County

The Fun Zone at Balboa (see Newport Harbor, page 87)

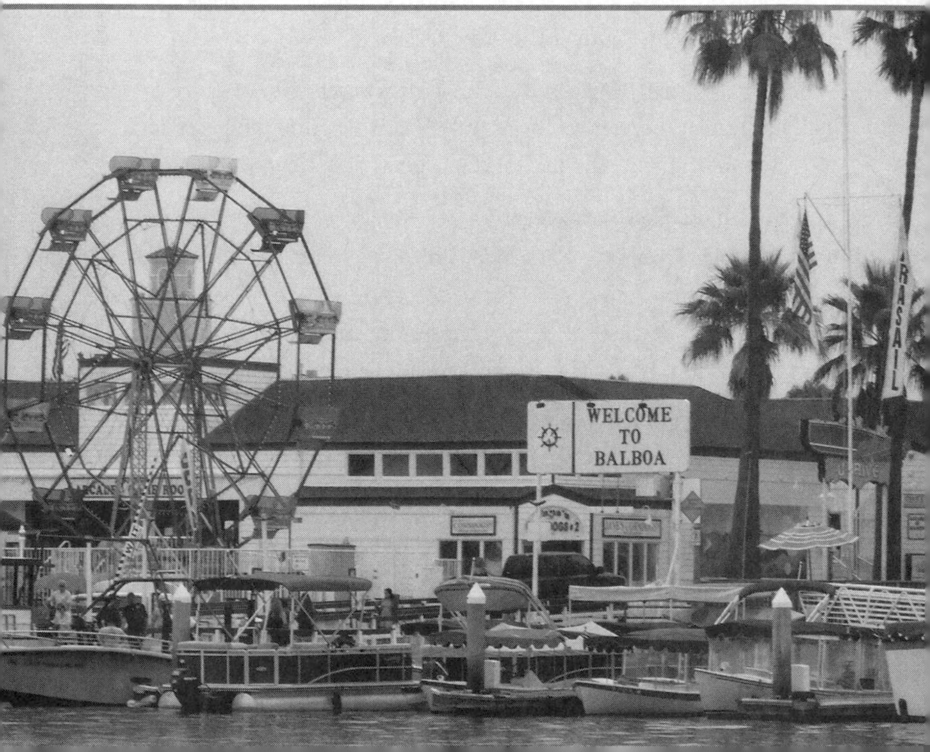

DANA POINT HARBOR AND BABY BEACH

Dana Point

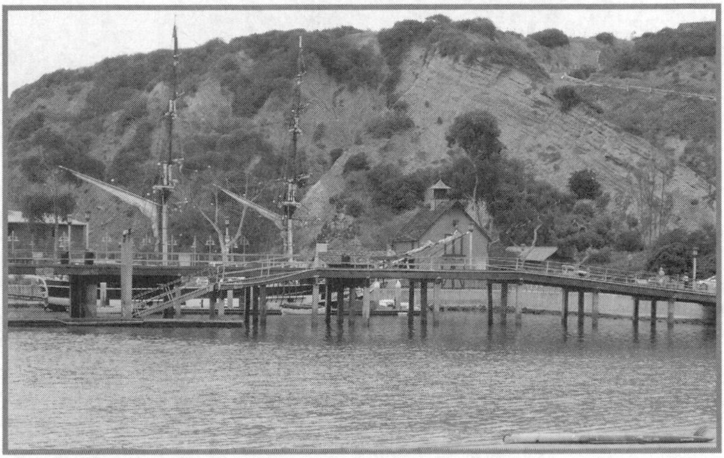

Baby Beach at Dana Point

OVERVIEW It was in 1835 when the famed sailing brig the *Pilgrim,* captained by a young Richard Henry Dana, first laid anchor in these waters. Dana, who later authored the nautical classic *Two Years Before the Mast,* described the local headland as "the only romantic spot in California." That was a hyperbolic claim for sure, but effective in the sense that the point still bears his name.

A century after the *Pilgrim*'s arrival, surfers laid claim to the point, heralding the long right-breaking wave as "Killer Dana." From the 1940s to the early 1960s, the point reigned as one of Southern California's legendary surf spots, but in 1966 the US Army Corps of Engineers began construction on a breakwater, building a jetty in the path of the former wave. The substantial loss to the surfing community was a boon to the boating community, as the breakwater set the stage for the creation of **Dana Point Harbor.**

.Officially opened in 1971, the harbor is a thriving commercial center with restaurants, shops, and two large basins full of dock space. There is also green space and the nonprofit **Ocean Institute.** As part of its program in marine education, the institute keeps a full-size, fully

Dana Point Harbor and Baby Beach

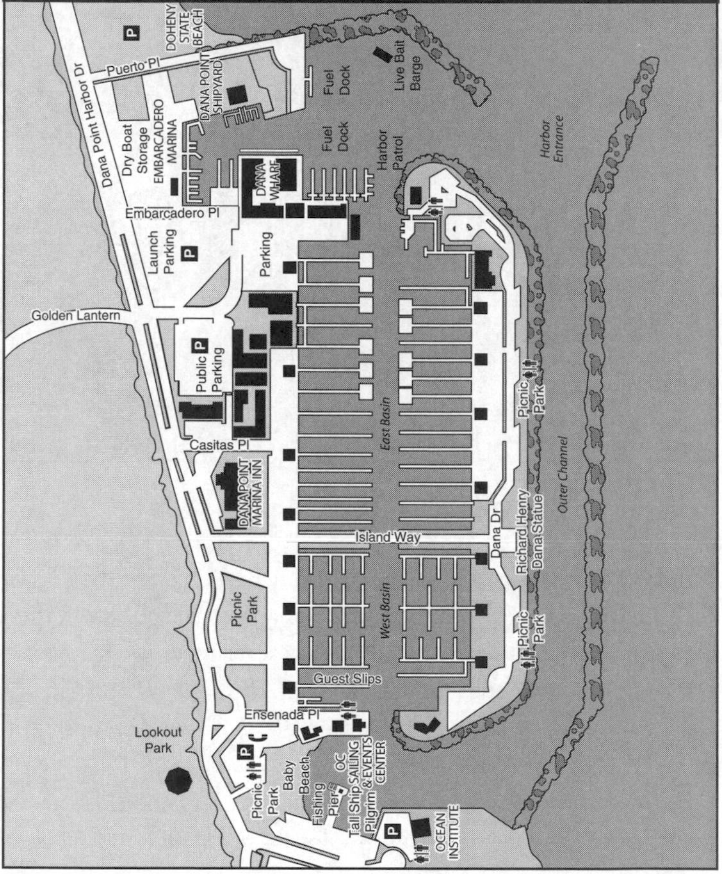

functioning replica of the *Pilgrim* docked on the west end of the harbor near Baby Beach. Scheduled tours of the vessel are available most of the year, the exception being late summer, when the *Pilgrim* takes to sea. The ship's return in September marks the occasion of the Tall Ships Festival, when the local fleet of historically significant vessels takes to the water, showing off their rigging, their seaworthiness, and their cannons.

Besides being home to the *Pilgrim*, **Baby Beach** is also a popular destination for paddlers. The calm conditions are perfect for novice paddlers, although more experienced paddlers may appreciate the abundance of free parking and the hassle-free launch. It's common to see a few pricey carbon race boards in the parking lot—owned by folks who don't want their expensive wares banged up in some gravelly shore break. The beach, managed by OC Parks, also has picnic tables, restroom facilities, and plenty of shady lawn space for keeping one's board out of the sun. **Westwind Sailing,** just to the left of the beach, offers courses in SUP instruction and fitness.

WHERE TO PADDLE Unlike Newport Harbor (see page 87), which was created by an estuary, man-made Dana Point is predictably gridlike, and navigating the harbor is fairly simple. From Baby Beach, heading south past the *Pilgrim* takes paddlers to the outer channel (just inside the breakwater). As you paddle south and east, the length of the outer channel leads you to the harbor entrance. At this point, paddlers may want to continue counterclockwise to the inner channel and circle back to Baby Beach. This route leads through the two major basins of docked space before returning to the launch point.

Those seeking a longer paddle may continue past the breakwater and into the open water. **Doheny State Beach** lies immediately beyond the harbor mouth, making a combination tour–surf session possible. (See "A SoCal SUS Sampler," page 180, for rules regarding stand-up surfing at Doheny.) If you simply want to paddle in the open water, pass the red bell-shaped marker that denotes the submerged Crawfish Rock; then continue along the line of buoys that parallel the coast toward Capistrano Beach. The buoys, essentially boundary markers for boats coming out of the harbor, make for a perfect paddling course.

Between 1 and 2 miles south of the harbor are a series of reefs—typically called "Capo reefs," as in Capistrano—and kelp paddies. During large surf events and storms, the reefs can actually produce breaking waves, but most days they remain calm. (With moderate-size surf, the underwater reefs may allow for the formation of cresting, nonbreaking waves.)

The kelp paddies are home to a number of game fish, including white sea bass, making this area popular with fishermen (check **danawharf.com/fishing** for more information) and deepwater divers. I wouldn't recommend combining this paddle with a dive or fishing expedition, however. For those wanting to fish or to surf the local reefs (recommended only for skilled stand-up paddlers with some local knowledge), launching at Doheny or Capistrano Beach is a better option.

DIRECTIONS AND PARKING From Pacific Coast Highway, head west on Green Lantern Drive. Continue 0.3 mile and then turn left on Cove Road. After 0.2 mile, turn right on Dana Point Harbor Drive. There is free parking in the lot on the left.

CONDITIONS AND HAZARDS They don't call it Baby Beach for nothing—this is a very user-friendly launch. But it's not by accident that Dana Point is a popular sailing spot. The area seems to be a magnet for afternoon sea breezes, so consider this particularly when venturing out of the harbor and toward Capistrano Beach. Your trip home will head directly into the prevailing winds.

RENTALS AND LESSONS **Dana Point Jet Ski and Kayak Center** (34671 Puerto Place; 949-661-4947, **danapointjetski.com**) rents SUP boards for $15 per hour and $40 for 4 hours. **Westwind Sailing** (34451 Ensenada Place; 949-923-2215, **westwindsailing.com**) offers a variety of courses that teach ocean safety, fitness, and paddling technique.

OCEAN INSTITUTE Offers opportunities for hands-on marine-science education. The Tall Ships Festival and the *Pilgrim* are the other big draws. (24200 Dana Point Harbor Drive; 949-496-2274, **ocean-institute.org**.)

LOCAL BURRITO After a good morning workout, head over to **Las Golondrinas** (34069 Doheny Park Road, Capistrano Beach; 949-240-8659, **lasgolondrinas.biz**) and try their nopalitos burrito. Tender cactus leaves are cooked up *machaca*-style with eggs and cheese. Pour a bit of their homemade salsa on top, and you're in for a rare treat.

Laguna Beach

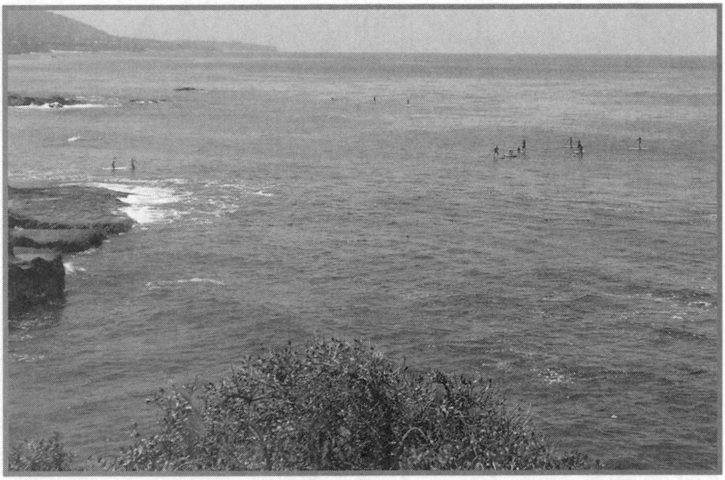

Paddlers near Fisherman's Cove in Laguna Beach

OVERVIEW In the summer of 2007, I met a man who was planning to open a surf shop in North Laguna. It seemed like a bold idea, starting a retail surf business outside the realm of touristy downtown. Because surf shops in Laguna Beach seem to survive more on the basis of T-shirt sales and rentals than on surfboard sales, I casually suggested that he might try to sell stand-up boards in his shop. Quite unexpectedly, the man browbeat me, told me I didn't know what I was talking about, and claimed that SUP boards, designated as watercraft, would soon be illegal to launch at local beaches.

I can't remember the name of that surf shop—it closed after six months—but today there are three active SUP shops in Laguna Beach, as well as rental companies, an outfit offering SUP tours, and plenty of SUP yoga classes.

Obviously, it's perfectly legal to launch paddleboards in the coves of Laguna, but the rising popularity of the sport has created some controversy. Concerns have been raised because Laguna beaches become crowded in the summer, and having swimmers and paddlers, particularly those new to the sport, in close vicinity creates safety issues. There are no outright SUP bans, but some nominal restrictions exist,

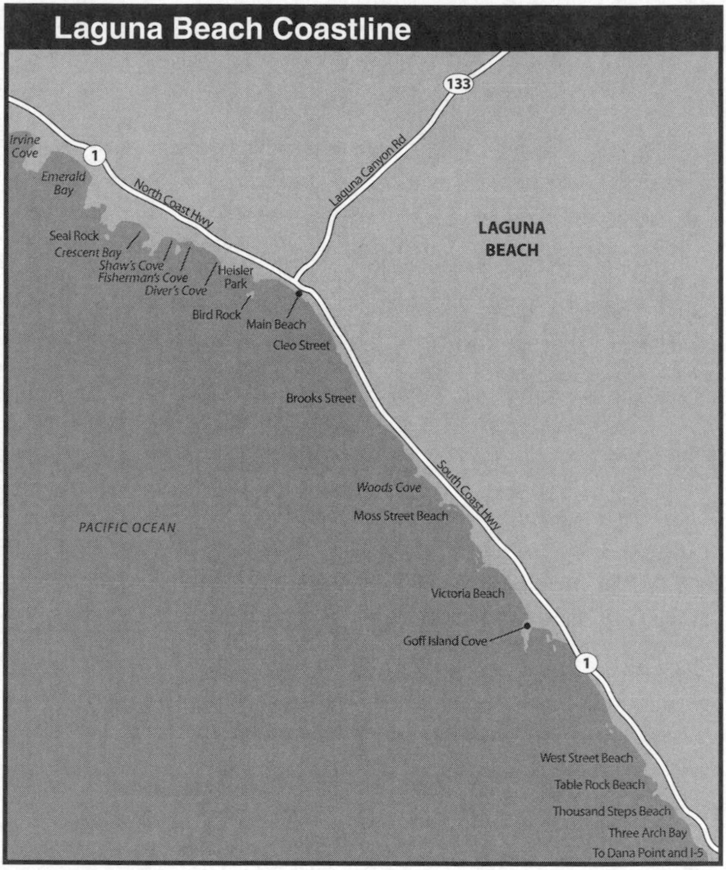

particularly on busy summer weekends. If a large number of swimmers is present, lifeguards may ask paddlers to stay outside the surf zone after launching. At certain coves, the lifeguards may direct paddlers to launch at a specific section of the beach—where there are the fewest swimmers, where the surf is the smallest, or both. Generally, the city lifeguards are helpful, willing to assist novice paddlers through the surf, and more concerned about safety than enforcing restrictions.

Although an SUP trip to Laguna Beach may involve dealing with crowds, traffic, and parking hassles, it's definitely worth it. Laguna is a great place to paddle. The city has 27 (!) coves scattered along

5.8 miles of picturesque coastline. Just outside the coves, a network of kelp paddies flourishes with sea life. Craggy rock formations line the coast, providing refuge to an array of birds (cormorants, pelicans, and seagulls are the most common), as well as, in one particular spot, a small colony of sea lions. Dolphin sightings are frequent, and migratory whales can be spotted within 200 yards of the shore. Because of its particular geography, the waters of Laguna Beach are less exposed to the elements than many other Orange County beaches. Although waves and wind can be a factor here, Laguna has plenty of calm, glassy days—days that any chamber of commerce would yearn for, days when the coastline is so ideally picturesque that it doesn't seem real.

Of course, there's nothing fake about the marine life in Laguna Beach. In 2012 the city was declared a state marine reserve, making the waters near shore a no-take zone from Irvine Cove to Treasure Island Beach. This was bad news for local fishermen, but it was a boon for nature lovers. My unscientific survey of the local beaches has revealed a dramatic increase in the fish populations. Coves where there used to be only garibaldi (protected statewide) now teem with schools of silver surf perch, calico bass, opaleye, and various forms of rockfish. Sightings of leopard sharks, halibut, and sheepshead are also common. The seeding of the local kelp beds also has helped in the creation of habitat space. In the last three years, encouraged by cool water and mild, sunny winters, these underwater forests have grown immensely, forming a protective barrier along much of the city's coastline.

WHERE TO PADDLE As I said before, crowds are an issue in Laguna Beach. It helps to have a strategy and a bit of local knowledge before trying to paddle these waters. Considering parking, traffic, and beach access, the two most favorable areas to launch are (1) in one of North Laguna's four accessible coves and (2) along the narrow strand that lies to the south of Main Beach (between Cleo and Brooks Streets).

NORTH LAGUNA

THE ADJOINING BEACHES of **Crescent Bay, Shaw's Cove, Fisherman's Cove,** and **Divers Cove** all offer excellent opportunities for launching

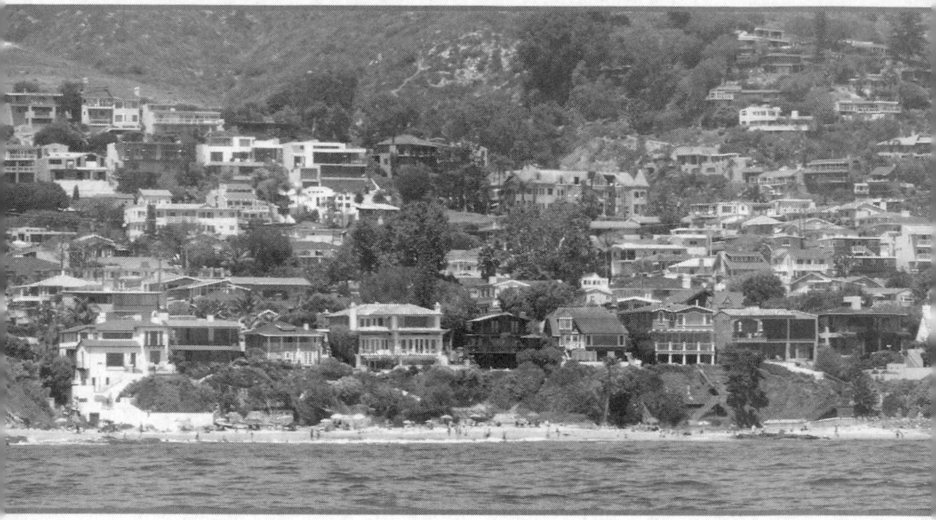

Shaw's Cove in Laguna Beach

SUP boards. Of these beaches, Crescent Bay is the most exposed to the surf, and Fisherman's Cove and Divers Cove tend to be the most protected—although launching at Fisherman's Cove during high tide can be tricky.

Scenic **Seal Rock** is the most common offshore destination from any of these coves. It's easy to see why the prominent rock with its eponymous, er, sea lions is a popular with paddlers. Park your board in the kelp-laden water outside the rock, and you'll be able to observe the colony of barking and waddling pinnipeds as they dive in and out of the water. On clear days, look for bubbles rising from the depths. You should be able to spy on the agile creatures as they dart back and forth under water, marking their territory and feasting on schools of small fish. When the weather cooperates, the waters outside Seal Rock afford nice views of the city and its rolling hillsides, as well as views of the weathered sandstone cliffs between Crescent Bay and Emerald Bay.

Paddling north of the rock takes you to the otherwise inaccessible beaches of **Emerald Bay** and **Irvine Cove.** These are two of the few remaining private beaches in Southern California. The stately cliffs of these coves are lined with some of the area's priciest real estate, fostering a tight-knit community of budding billionaires. Out on the water, particularly on summer weekends, Emerald Bay attracts a fleet of luxurious yachts, so if you come across one, don't hesitate to paddle up and ask for your share of the Grey Poupon.

Just south of Fisherman's Cove and stretching down to Main Beach, one finds the most substantial kelp growths in the city. Although SUPing through the paddies can be a bit sticky, it can also be quite rewarding. Stay to the leeward side of the kelp beds to find smooth, clean-textured water and amazing deepwater views. (I'm not sure about the scientific factors, but the water just beyond the kelp offers the most clarity for deepwater visibility.) The sight of the golden tendrils of kelp, reaching down into the depths, is quite mesmerizing. On nice days, it's tempting to park out on the paddies and enjoy the gentle motion of the water as it rolls through the floating forest of kelp. For this reason, the kelp beds off **Heisler Park** are a popular spot for SUP yoga classes. Students often brace or stabilize their boards with the long strands of seaweed before performing poses.

Inside of the kelp beds and closer to Heisler Park is the popular **Rockpile** surf break. The name was not given by accident—several craggy heads and reefs lie above and below the surface (depending on tide). On small surf days, this is also an apt location to view marine life. It's impossible to miss the bright-orange garibaldi that frequent these waters, but on closer inspection, you might also play witness to lurking reef fish, fast-moving schools of groupers, or even spiny lobsters.

Directly offshore, at the south end of Heisler, is **Bird Rock,** so named for its ever-present congregation of cormorants, seagulls, and pelicans. At medium to high tide, it's possible to paddle inside of Bird Rock. If you do, hope for a bit of sea breeze, because the guano stink can be pretty intense.

South of Bird Rock is the open strand of **Main Beach.** In the summer months, lifeguards will warn you away from paddling too close to shore here, but they'll generally assist you if you want to beach or launch along this crowded section.

SOUTH OF MAIN BEACH

SOUTH OF THE Hotel Laguna (it's the big white building), from Cleo Street to Brooks Street, is a narrow stretch of beach popular with young surfers, skimboarders, and swimmers. A couple of shops here rent SUP boards, so paddleboarders frequent this stretch as well.

Although this beach is wide open and less quaint than the coves of North Laguna, it's a good starting point to head south to scenic **Moss Cove, Woods Cove, Victoria Beach,** and **Goff Island Cove.** This final beach, directly in front of the Montage Hotel, offers some of the finest snorkeling in the area. From Oak Street, it's about 1.5 miles along the rocky coast down to Goff Island. This is a nice outing; the waters near the Montage are generally calm, clear, and perfect for paddling. However, launching at Goff Island Cove requires a long walk through the hotel grounds to reach the sand. I would recommend making it a destination rather than a starting point.

Those who don't desire a long paddle may be content exploring some of the offshore reefs at Brooks Street and the kelp beds that extend from Oak Street to Cleo Street (not as thick as in North Laguna, but still worth a look).

Stand-up surfers are commonly found along the breaks in front of the Pacific Edge Hotel, Oak Street, and Thalia Street, but I don't recommend SUPing at these breaks unless you have a decent amount of surfing experience and some local knowledge. Crowds of prone surfers will be prevalent along this stretch; also, the waves tend to close out quickly and often break close to shore (not ideal for larger boards). In the summer, particularly when kids' surf schools are in the water, lifeguards will instruct SUPers to stay outside of the surf zone.

WHALE-WATCHING

IN THE LATE fall and early spring, migrating gray whales pass through the local waters. They seem to take a course directly around

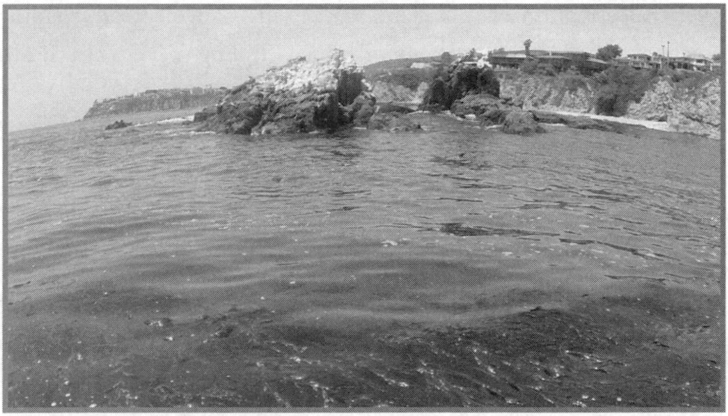

Seal Rock and its barrier of kelp

Dana Point, staying tight to the coast of Laguna Beach. Sightings are frequent, and several whale-watching charters troll the local waters with boatloads of tourists. Paddlers who want to get up close and personal with gray whales probably have to paddle just 200–500 yards offshore for the opportunity. Without the range or the sonar equipment of the commercial boats, paddlers are advised to keep an eye out for whale charters. This is the easiest way to find whales—either from shore or on the water. Look for the slow-moving boats, and the whales will often be nearby.

Behemoth blue whales also pass through the region, although rarely close to shore. A crew of paddlers launches in the coves of North Laguna and then navigates about 2 miles offshore in order to watch and photograph blue whales. It's a somewhat substantial commitment of time and energy, but the experience of encountering one of the world's largest mammals in the open ocean is absolutely extraordinary.

DIRECTIONS There are only two entry points into Laguna Beach: **Pacific Coast Highway** and **Laguna Canyon Road.** If you're arriving from the north, avoid busy Laguna Canyon and take the PCH to one of the points in North Laguna. Obviously, when taking the PCH from the south end of town, the beaches south of Main Beach will be your easiest destination. If you arrive via Laguna Canyon Road, heading toward North Laguna will generally mean dealing with less traffic.

Directions to Crescent Bay Beach: From I-405, head south on I-73 and exit at MacArthur Boulevard. Drive south on MacArthur for 2.7 miles. When MacArthur ends, turn left on PCH and continue south for 5.9 miles. Once in Laguna, take the second right onto Cliff Drive. Follow Cliff Drive about 500 feet to the access for Crescent Bay.

PARKING AND LAUNCHING Timing is everything. Because parking is such an issue in Laguna, paddlers will do best to arrive at the beach early in the morning on summer days (and particularly summer weekends), when the water is typically calmer and the beaches less crowded.

All the beaches I've profiled above have nearby street parking and either stairs or ramps to access the beach. In North Laguna, Cliff Drive runs parallel to the beaches of Crescent Bay, Shaw's Cove, Fisherman's Cove, and Divers Cove. Crescent Bay has two access points, one at Circle Way (off Cliff Drive) and one at Chiquita Street. The stairway to Shaw's Cove is at the bottom of Fairview Street. The stairs to both Fisherman's Cove and Divers Cove are on Cliff Drive just south of Beverly Street. Free street parking is available along this stretch, and then metered parking south of Divers Cove where Cliff Drive runs adjacent to Heisler Park.

If you can't find a place to park near one of the beach-access points, it may be best to unload your board close to the walkway and then find a spot. There is no perfect algorithm: Just try to beat the crowds and use common sense—and always pay the meters, which are closely watched by the local parking-enforcement team.

Street parking is also available on the ocean side of PCH between Cleo Street and Oak Street—this includes a very limited supply of free parking and some metered parking. Again, arrive early and be vigilant about feeding the meters.

CONDITIONS AND HAZARDS Laguna tends to have relatively calmer conditions than the beaches to the north and south. That doesn't mean, though, that wind and waves won't be a factor. During large southwest swells, launching at the coves in Laguna may be tricky or even dangerous. The afternoon wind tends to be stronger near Seal Rock and less prevalent in and around Main Beach.

Crowds are a factor in the summer. September and October tend to have nice weather and small beach crowds.

FACILITIES Restrooms and showers are available at Crescent Bay Beach, as well as at the north end of Main Beach.

RENTALS AND LESSONS **Bliss Paddle Yoga** (949-529-4242, **paddleboardbliss.com**) is a mother–daughter company that began in Laguna Beach and has now expanded to Newport Beach and San Diego. They offer rentals, demonstrations, and yoga every weekend at Divers Cove. I recommend the Bliss folks to anyone wanting to get into SUP or SUP yoga. Go to their website to check out their busy schedule of events and their own line of SUP products.

La Vida Laguna (1257 S. Coast Highway; 949-275-7544, **lavidalaguna.com**), a full-service outdoor-activity company, offers SUP tours out of Fisherman's Cove. Their guided tours, which include a trip to Seal Rock, are 2 hours long and cost $100.

Brawner Boards (1101 S. Coast Highway; 949-480-7649, **brawnerboards.com**) is a full-service board shop on PCH just north of Brooks Street. SUP rentals run $40 for 2 hours and $60 for 4 hours. They also offer private, semiprivate, and group lessons.

CA Surf N' Paddle (695 S. Coast Highway; 949-497-1423, **casurfshop.com**) rents SUP boards for $25 per hour and $50 per day. They're affiliated with the Costa Azul Surf Shop, on PCH near Cleo Street.

LOCAL BURRITO This is an easy one: **La Sirena Grill.** These guys make healthy Mexican food that's also amazingly delicious. Although you'd probably be happy with just about anything they serve, I suggest forgoing what's on the menu and simply asking for the unlisted calamari burrito. Trust me on this. There are two locations in Laguna Beach: 347 Mermaid St. (949-497-8226, **lasirenagrill.com/lagunabeach**) and 30862 S. Coast Highway (949-499-2301, **lasirenagrill.com/southlaguna**).

Crystal Cove State Park

Laguna Beach–Corona Del Mar

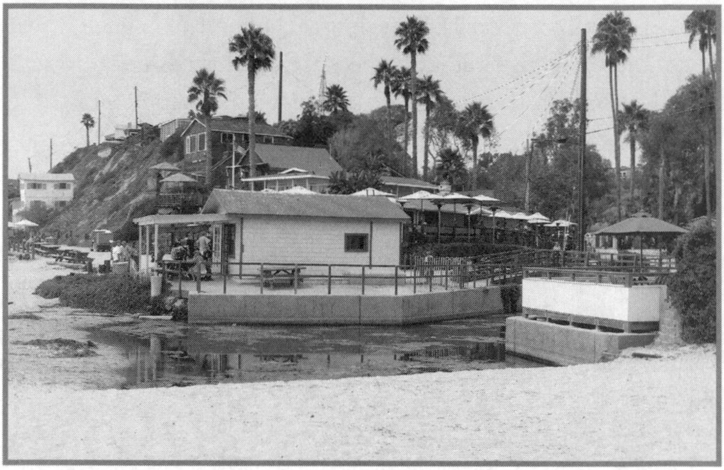

Cottages in the Historic District at Crystal Cove State Park

OVERVIEW Stretching from the north end of Laguna Beach to the southern border of Corona Del Mar, Crystal Cove State Park offers 3.2 miles of coastal paradise—wide, sandy beaches; tidepools; surf breaks; deepwater reefs; and picturesque cliffs. Because of its long, unobstructed strand, this beach park is popular with walkers and runners. For most of the park's span, steep seaside cliffs block the view and the noise of nearby Coast Highway. Spending an afternoon here can reinvigorate one's notions of the possibilities of Southern California life. As you relax in the sand, it's easy to recall a simpler time before the local hills and canyons were graded, parceled, and commoditized—a time when the coast was wild, abalone grew like apples on the local reefs, and the love of salt water trumped just about every other concern.

The good news is that the salt water is still here and, in some ways, still as magnificent and restorative as ever. Even though the abalones are few and far between, there is a healthy population of spiny lobsters and a recently invigorated population of reef fish, along with bottlenose dolphins, pinnipeds, and the occasional migrating whale.

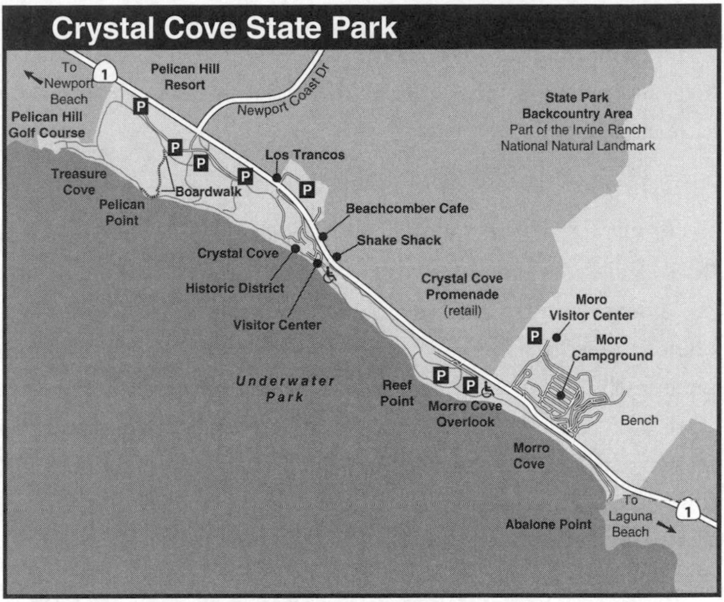

WHERE TO PADDLE For the paddleboarder, access to these waters requires only admission to the state park. There are four entrance points, but the most convenient SUP access is at El Morro. (*Note:* Due to a recording error, California State Parks refers to the region as El Moro or Moro Cove, but the correct spelling—and the one used by locals—is El Morro, with two *R*'s.)

From the parking lot, walk under Coast Highway through a tunnel. (This is also the point where El Morro Creek flows to the ocean. For most of the year, however, the water stops short of its goal and remains in a stagnant pool to the left of the walkway.) Once on the shore, feel free to launch anywhere along the sandy beach, maybe trying to find a spot with the fewest swimmers. Except for a couple of submerged rocks about 100 yards north of the tunnel, the entire stretch of beach at El Morro is sandy-bottomed, so you have plenty of options for launching and landing. The surf tends to break close to shore, but on most days you can push through the break to the relative calm of deep water. It's not a terribly difficult launch, except during large south-swell events.

On these days, you may want to leave your paddleboard on the sand and try your hand at bodysurfing. If you have any questions, there are lifeguards in towers during the summer months and roving lifeguards in vehicles throughout the entire year.

OPTION 1

INTREPID PADDLERS WILL want to make the trip to isolated **Irvine Cove.** Paddle south from the tunnel, down the beach, and toward the prominent point that marks the border of the state park. The oft-photographed headland—with its painterly cliffs and a signature knoll in the shape of camel's hump—is what gives El Morro ("the point") its name. The first half-mile of the paddle follows an open section of beach. There used to be trailer homes along this strand, but they were removed in 2006, and now all that stands here is a three-story concrete-and-glass lifeguard facility. (The building looks like a cross between an airport control tower and a car wash.)

As you near the cliff, you might see a few surfers lined up near the rocks. Waves break a little farther from shore here, but not dramatically so, and it's easy to stay in deep water and out of the break. Past the first turn in the point, a few rocky coves nestle inside an exposed reef that forms the extreme edge of the headland. The view of the cliffs here is dramatic and somehow unexpected—most of this rocky shoreline is visible only from the water. Although the water remains deep even near the cliff's edge, paddling in close proximity to the rocks can be a bit challenging due to wave refraction. This is particularly true on south-wind days, when your board may feel a bit like a cork in a bathtub, tossing back and forth. Except on the calmest days, it may behoove you to stay outside of the rock cove, enjoying the larger view of the cliffs and the hills of Laguna Beach.

If you're game, continue paddling all the way around the point. Once you've passed the home of land baroness Joan Irvine Smith (it's the one with the pagoda perched on the edge of the cliff), you've reached the waters of Irvine Cove. The inlet, protected by the aforementioned cliffs, is a fantastic snorkeling spot. Among the highlights

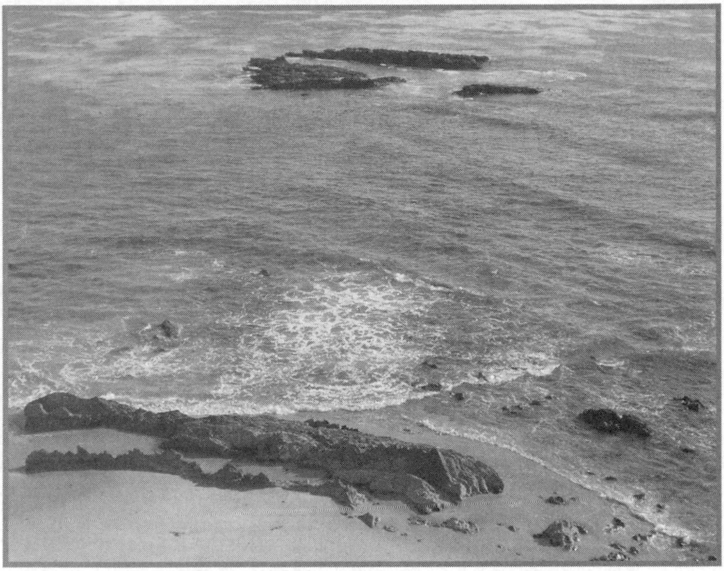

Reef Point at Crystal Cove State Park

here is a substantial population of bat rays; take a chance to spy on them as they launch from the sandy bottom and soar gracefully through the water. The rays look menacing but are harmless and, unless provoked, mind their own business. The local sea lion population, however, is quite territorial, so expect to be the center of attention if you paddle or swim into the west side of the cove. The colony is neither dangerously aggressive nor mean-spirited, but they are very attached to their rookery and will remain nearby, keeping a careful eye the entire time you're in *their* waters.

To finish the journey, paddle the rest of the way to the beach and then luxuriate in the sand on one of the most exclusive beaches in Southern California. Bask in the sun, look up at the collection of $20 million homes, and be thankful you don't have to pay the mortgage. The only access to this beach is via the water—the community is private and the beach locked in by cliffs, making for perfectly uncrowded conditions.

OPTION 2

A LESS DEMANDING trip would be to paddle up the beach toward **Reef Point.** This option may be particularly advantageous in the summer, when prevailing west winds can pick up in the afternoon. If the wind becomes a factor, your return trip will be downwind. There is also a healthy barrier of kelp along the shore, making for smoother paddling conditions.

From the tunnel, paddle toward Corona Del Mar. It's about 0.5 mile to the rocks that mark Scotchman's Cove. This first stretch is wide open aside from two minor submerged reefs, and the kelp forest runs parallel to the beach, only about 75 yards offshore. Scotchman's Cove is a shorter, rocky-bottomed span. On calm days, you'll be able to paddle in over the sea grass and catch glimpses of some of the local marine life. Though rarely seen in the daylight, a significant population of spiny lobsters lives in these waters. From September to March, the collection of buoys found here signals the presence of submerged lobster pots managed by commercial fishermen.

Reef Point lies on the far end of Scotchman's Cove. The rocky spits form the barrier between Scotchman's and crescent-shaped Abalone Cove. Two exposed rocks, split by a narrow channel, rest about 50 yards offshore and mark the outer edge of the point. At higher tides (say, above 3 feet), you can paddle inside the exposed rocks, but when doing so, be careful of submerged obstacles and incoming surf. Potential surf breaks lie on both sides of the point, so use the presence of surfers—and their relative position—to gauge the possibility of waves.

The waters around Pelican Point also offer some of the best snorkeling opportunities in the state park. If you're an accomplished diver, you may want to ditch your board for a while and explore the steep craggy surface along the channel of the split rock. Otherwise, simply paddling over the shallow expanse of sea grass affords views of the resident marine life. There are also sea lions here; while not territorial like the ones in Irvine Cove, they may pay a visit if you're fishing. (Unlike in Laguna, fishing and spearfishing are legal in the state park.)

If you paddle around the outside of Reef Point, expect to navigate through a thick section of kelp before reaching the open waters of **Abalone Point.** For a longer outing, paddle the length of Abalone Cove and outside a section of rocky shore until you reach the open strand at **Crystal Cove.** The beach that gives the state park its name is home to a collection of rustic beach cottages. California State Parks refers to this as the "historic district." Some of the cottages are restored and available for overnight stays; others are boarded up and left to stand as monuments to the ragtag group of folks who lived in a commune here from the 1920s to the 1990s.

As at El Morro, the beach is sandy here, making it easy to land and enjoy the beach and the local amenities. Although the historic district has a bit of a theme park quality, it's still a beautiful beach, and investigation of some of the still-unrestored cottages might give one a true impression of what it was like to live here.

For the hungry, the **Beachcomber Restaurant** serves breakfast, lunch, and dinner, starting at 7 a.m. Just up the stairs toward Coast Highway, the **Crystal Cove Shake Shack** serves up date shakes, smoothies, and casual food with a nice view daily from 7 a.m. to 9 p.m.

DIRECTIONS AND PARKING Crystal Cove State Park is off Pacific Coast Highway between Corona Del Mar and Laguna Beach. Access the El Morro Canyon entrance via Pacific Coast Highway (0.6 mile north and 2.6 miles south of Corona Del Mar). Turn at the light at School/State Park Road (there's only one way you can go) and continue behind El Morro School to the entrance kiosk. From the entrance, continue down the big hill to the day-use parking area. Try to park as close to the tunnel as possible. The day-use fee for the state park is $15; annual passes cost $195.

RESTRICTIONS As of this writing, it's legal to launch SUP boards in Crystal Cove State Park, but lifeguards may enforce restrictions when crowds or large surf pose a safety risk. As a rule, try to launch and land away from swimmers.

CONDITIONS AND HAZARDS During large south swells, robust waves break close to shore at El Morro. On most days, the surf will be larger at Reef Point and El Morro Point. Paddlers keen on making the trip to Irvine Cove should know that once they pass El Morro, there is no beach access until they reach the cove. West winds may be prominent in the afternoon but are less strong than at the beaches in Newport, Huntington, and Long Beach.

The cliff at El Morro

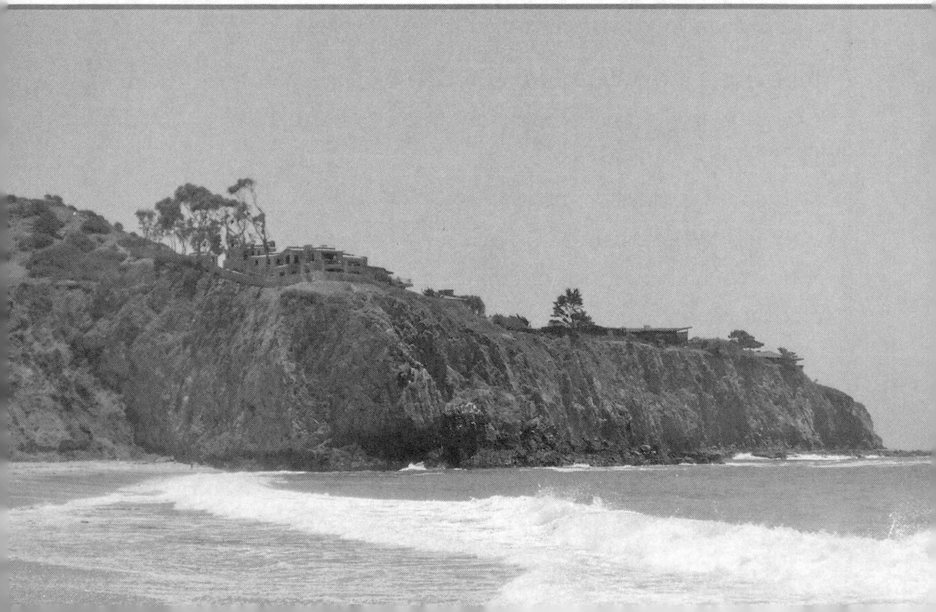

Newport Harbor

Newport Beach

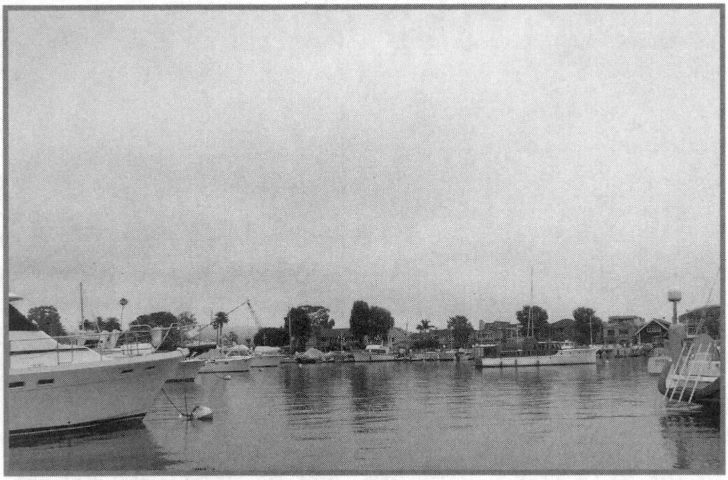

Paddling path through the moorings

OVERVIEW Bordered by Pacific Coast Highway and the Balboa Peninsula, Newport Harbor is an extensive waterway that contains a network of channels, bridges, and small islands. Before the development of Newport Beach, the entire area was a bog—a wetland inside a narrow sand spit—just waiting to be transformed by land owners and speculators. The original purpose of the harbor may have been commercial, but today the area is mostly residential, a real estate gold mine known for its yacht clubs, waterfront mansions, large-windowed restaurants, and more expensive pleasure boats than you can point a stick at (or a paddle, for that matter).

In the summer, tourists flock to the area to sun on the beaches (mostly on the ocean side), revel in the bars (on the beaches and the bay), and eat frozen bananas (more on that later). In December, residents put Christmas lights on their boats and parade around the harbor, fueled by cocktails and canapés. The rest of the year is divided up nicely by USC football and the Newport to Ensenada Yacht Race.

Newport Harbor isn't just a place; it's a place with a lifestyle few can afford. But that doesn't mean there isn't any diversity on the

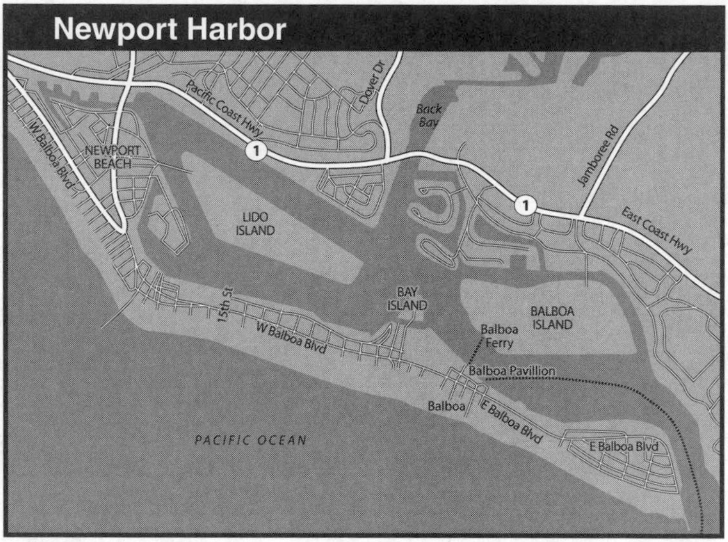

water. (Not all of the harbor's denizens subscribe to *The Robb Report.*) On breezy days, diminutive Lido and Laser sailboats dart out of the public launches and basic Duffy electric boats are rented by the hour; near the breakwater are several fishing charters, whale-tour boats, and the ferry to Catalina.

The protected waters also offer plenty of opportunities for paddling. Not only is the area user-friendly and accessible, it's quite scenic in its own way—a wonderland of pricey real estate and nautical delights. New boats, old boats, carefully restored boats, and rust-bucket boats all add to the character of the place. There are also plenty of waterways, inlets, and small passages. One could spend months exploring the ins and outs of this bay. I've listed one basic paddle, but if you take the time to explore, there are plenty of opportunities to find new routes and new launch sites.

WHERE TO PADDLE The streets of the Newport Peninsula are easy to navigate. **Balboa Boulevard,** the primary artery, runs the length of the strand, and the intersecting numbered streets descend in order as you drive farther away from Pacific Coast Highway. (First Street is a few blocks away from the Balboa Pavilion. Lettered and various named streets follow.)

Paddle Power, a kayak-and-SUP shop, rests on the corner of Balboa and 15th Street. One short block away, between the Legion Hall and a row of private homes, are a public dock and a small beach to launch from. On most days (perhaps excluding summer weekends), it's easy to find metered parking near the launch site, and you'll find grass in front of the Legion Hall and a bit of sand near the dock in case you need to put your board down before gearing up to go paddling.

You can launch off the dock, but there are often folks fishing there, so it may be easier to launch in the small space to the right of the dock. Once in the water, head right and southward toward Balboa Island; this will give you a broader view of what the harbor has to offer. From the launch, it's roughly 2 miles to the turnaround point at the **Balboa Pavilion.** This is also the site of the Balboa Ferry and close to the home of Balboa Island's world-famous frozen bananas, which were made even more famous after being featured on the TV show *Arrested Development.* I recommend watching an episode or two of the show before making the paddle. This will give you a bit of satiric insight to the culture of the area, and perhaps a few things to chuckle about as you glide through the water.

As you push away from the dock, you'll pass through a collection of mooring sites. The shores of **Lido Island** will be directly across the channel. After a half-mile, past the south end of Lido Island, is the largest open area of the harbor. Continue south past **Bay Island** (it's on the right—the small island with only a pedestrian bridge) and head down the peninsula. Once you pass Bay Island, Balboa Island will be on your left.

After a few minutes, the Balboa Ferry and the Pavilion come into view. The ferry has been carrying cars and passengers from the island to the peninsula for more than 80 years. It runs constantly all day and night, so you're sure to see it in operation. It doesn't move fast, but I would advise keeping your distance. As a paddler, you should have right-of-way over just about every vessel in the harbor, but probably not the ferry, a cross-channel vehicle. I'm pretty sure the ferry drivers are happy to steer out of your way . . . but do you really want them to?

I remember a trip on the ferry many years ago when a passenger was pushed as a prank by his friend, who probably didn't expect what happened next: The luckless fellow went into the water just as the ferry was pulling into the dock. Afraid that the guy might be crushed, the young ferry captain was about to put the controls in reverse. But before he could, an elderly man, appearing like a ghost out of a New England seafaring novel, cried *"Noooo!"* What the elderly man knew was that the ferry engines don't work in reverse—there are two engines, one on each end, and they only thrust. Therefore, putting the ferry in reverse would have activated the front engines nearest to the fallen man. Lucky for him, the young captain listened, and the man was able to swim clear under the dock.

This may be a story worth remembering if you want to paddle close to the ferry: The vessel may move slowly enough, it's highly visible, and it should be able to veer around you—but don't paddle in front of it thinking it will be able to stop.

Past the Balboa Pavilion, the harbor continues for more than a mile until it feeds into the open ocean. Head to the breakwater if you feel like a longer paddle, but if you've had enough or you have only so much time on your parking meter, turn back at the pavilion and retrace your route. You're bound to see a few things on the return trip that you missed on the way out.

DIRECTIONS AND PARKING From Pacific Coast Highway, follow Balboa Boulevard 1.6 miles and turn left onto 15th Street. Metered parking is available on both sides of the street for $1 per hour. The meters accept quarters or credit cards. Note that parking is suspended on Wednesday mornings for street sweeping. You may find free parking on West Bay Avenue, but be sure to check the streetside signs for hours and restrictions.

CONDITIONS AND HAZARDS Paddling here is generally accessible and safe. On most days, expect calm waters and easy paddling. Summer afternoons may tend to get a bit breezy, but chop is rarely an issue.

Weekends will find the waters crowded, as boats large and small make their way around the harbor and out to the ocean. Within the harbor, boats are restricted to slow speeds and generally not allowed to create a wake.

A weekly inside-the-harbor sailboat race is held on Friday evenings in the spring and summer. The holiday Boat Parade runs the week before Christmas. Plenty of crowds come for the evening festivities.

RENTALS **Paddle Power,** on the corner of 15th Street and Balboa Boulevard (949-675-1215, **paddlepowerh2o.com**), rents boards from 10 a.m. to 5:30 p.m. Monday–Friday, and from 9 a.m. to 5:30 p.m. Saturday and Sunday. Rates are $20 per hour and $75 per day. They also carry a large selection of boards and paddles.

LOCAL BURRITO Every local knows that **Bear Flag Fish Company** (3421 Via Lido; 949-673-3474, **newport.bearflagfishco.com**) concocts some of the best Mexican seafood on the planet. I recommend the ahi poke burrito. It's not on the regular menu, but order it once and your life will be forever changed.

Looking toward Pacific Coast Highway. The Back Bay is just beyond the bridge.

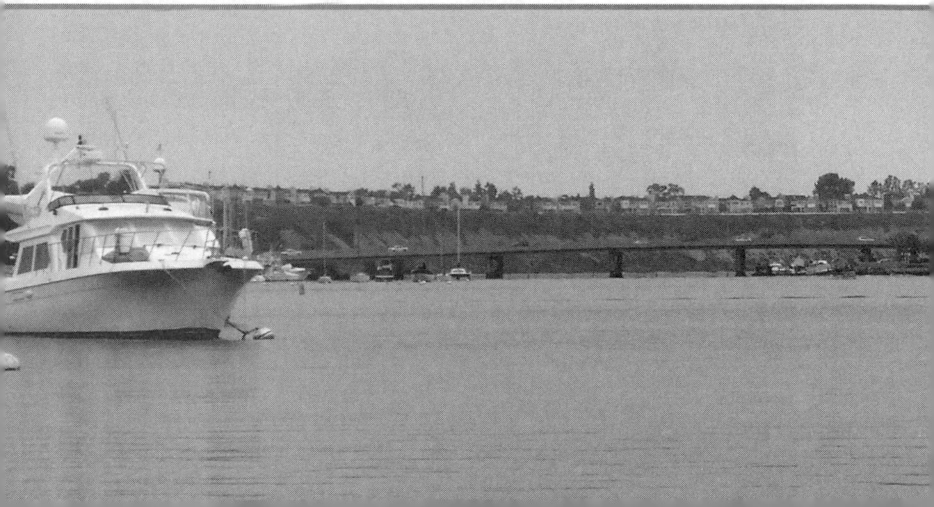

NEWPORT BACK BAY **Newport Beach**

(See map on page 88)

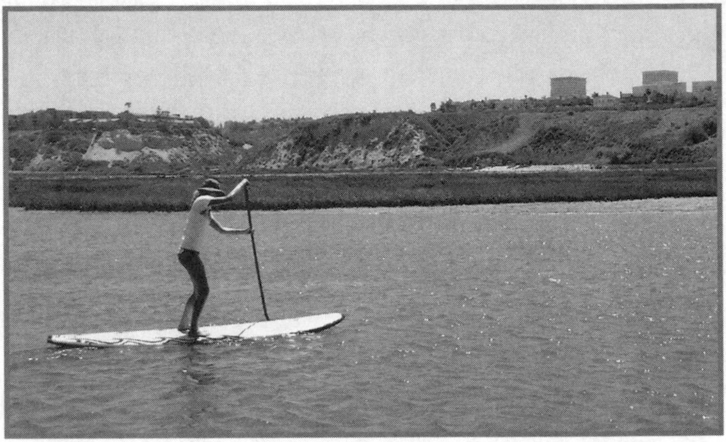

Paddling in front of the Newport Aquatic Center

OVERVIEW "Back Bay" is the colloquial term for the upper reaches of Newport Harbor. The shallow, cliff-lined, bird-rich waterway is one of the few remaining natural estuaries in Southern California. Consequently, the area is a nature preserve, completely open to all forms of paddling, except for a few restricted areas accessible only to rangers and permit holders. (The boundaries for paddlers without permits are clearly marked with signs. The off-limits areas tend to be in the shallow, reedy sections.)

If you desire a serene paddling experience over calm waters, replete with scenic surroundings and wildlife, then you'll find Back Bay more than suitable. If you desire a workout-based paddle, with plenty of space, turnaround markers, and other paddlers to gauge your speed against, again I would recommend Back Bay. The area offers plenty of calm, shallow water. Busy Pacific Coast Highway and the office towers of Newport Center are visible from the water, but it's easy to ignore their proximity and focus on the immediate scenery, the shorebirds, and the glassy stillness of the water. (Even the jets flying overhead shouldn't disturb you—local John Wayne Airport requires all departing jets to buffer their engine noise.) When paddling Back Bay, you may be in a fishbowl surrounded by suburbia, but suburbia is playing coy, telling you to focus on the avian wildlife and the painterly cliffs.

WHERE TO PADDLE The **Newport Aquatic Center** is the best place to access the Back Bay. Here you'll find plenty of free parking and a wide, sandy beach for launching. Of course, you won't be alone: At the Aquatic Center, SUP boards share the beach with outriggers, kayaks, sculls, and canoes. If you can paddle it, you'll find it here, but there is plenty of space for everyone.

From the beach, either paddle left and inland to the upper reaches of Back Bay, or right toward Pacific Coast Highway, along the channel and striking cliffs of **Dover Shores.** Paddlers going up the Back Bay have the option to head out nearly 2 miles into the estuary before turning around near the bridge at Jamboree. The paddle toward Pacific Coast Highway will be busier with boats—and, on weekends, the impressively fast outrigger crews—but this might be a better option in breezy conditions, as the prevailing wind comes in from the ocean and up the bay. The shorter paddle toward PCH doesn't explore as much of the estuary, but it still offers an opportunity to view nesting blue herons and take in the scenic (though decidedly not white) cliffs of Dover Shores.

Paddlers wanting to put in several miles of flat-water training can continue under PCH and then paddle the length of Newport Harbor (see previous profile). Paddlers have plenty of options here; just be sure not to pass the signs marking the limits of public access.

DIRECTIONS AND PARKING *From Pacific Coast Highway:* Turn onto Dover Drive (heading inland) and drive 0.7 mile. Turn right onto Westcliff Drive. After 0.3 mile, turn right onto Santiago Drive and then take the first left onto Polaris Drive. After 0.4 mile, pull into the Newport Aquatic Center parking lot, on your right.

From I-55: Follow the freeway until it ends and then turn left on 17th Street. Turn left on Dover Drive, then immediately turn right onto Westcliff Drive. Follow the directions above to the Newport Aquatic Center. There are also signs pointing the way.

RENTALS AND LESSONS SUP boards may be rented for $20 per hour at the **Newport Aquatic Center** (1 White Cliffs Drive; 949-626-7725, **newportaquaticcenter.com**). Lessons are available, as well as camps and tours; children younger than age 12 are required to wear life vests. Hours are 7 a.m.–5 p.m. Monday–Friday, 7 a.m.–4:15 p.m. Saturday and Sunday.

LOCAL BURRITO The friendly folks at **Los Primos** make the largest vegetarian burrito this side of the 5 Freeway. The Dr. Carlos Special—apparently named after a doctor who prescribed gluttony—is made with heaps of black beans, rice, iceberg lettuce, guacamole, Cheddar cheese, pico de gallo, salsa, and sour cream, all rolled up in two large overlapping flour tortillas. *It's not a burrito, it's a banquet.* Just the construction of this beast is a sight to behold. Have it for two meals or have it for three; either way, you get your $6.49 worth. (488 E. 17th St., #A106; 949-650-1486.)

Los Angeles County

The outer beach at Cabrillo (see page 101)

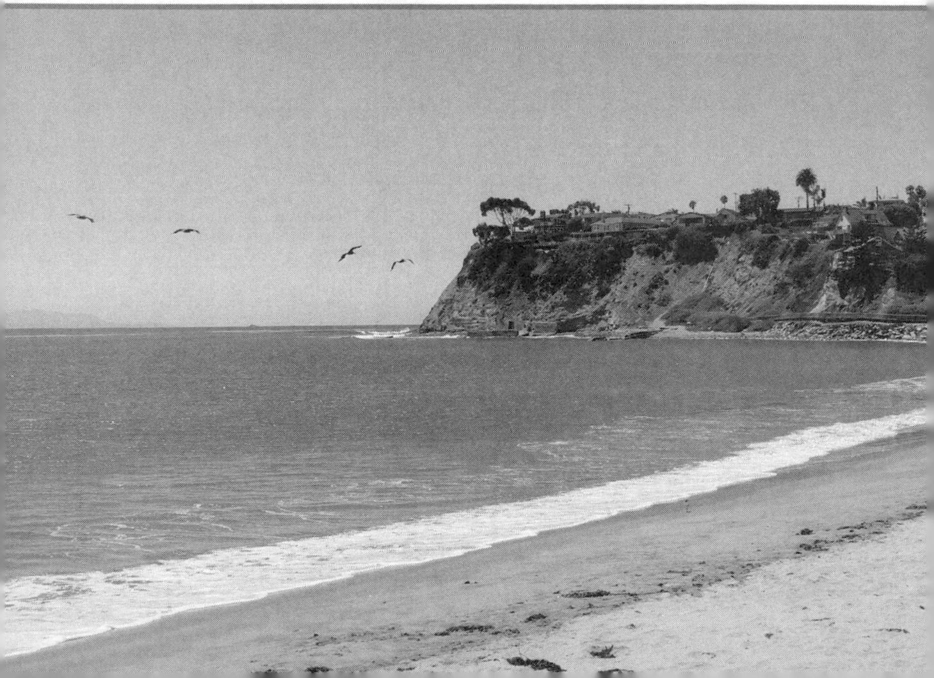

Belmont Shore Long Beach

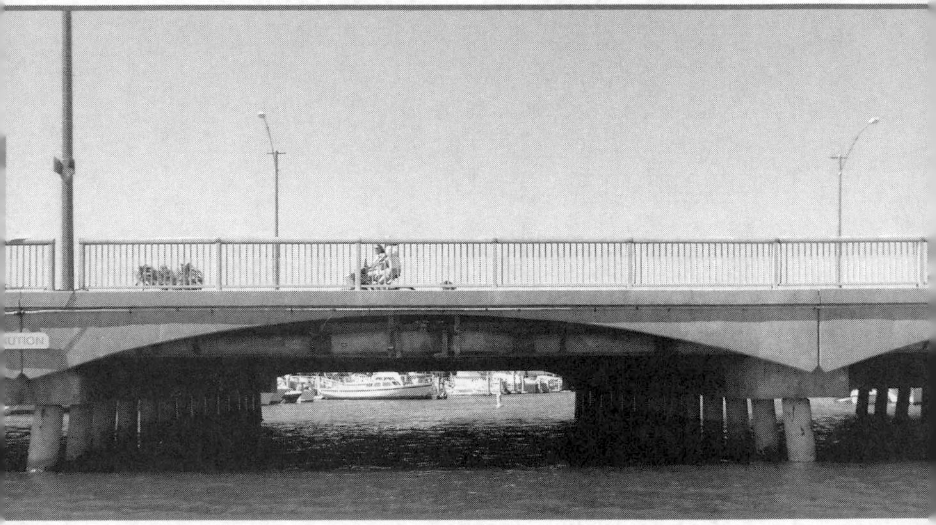

The Second Street Bridge

OVERVIEW A water-bound borough of Long Beach that lies just west of the Orange County border, Belmont Shore is a compact beach community that has become a haven for hip, young, and active adults. And why not? It's a great place to visit—and to live.

Between the grid of residential space, the main drag of **East Second Street** offers a variety of boutiquelike shops, bars, restaurants, and coffeehouses. Of course, like any popular beach town with narrow streets and compact neighborhoods, Belmont Shore suffers from traffic and parking woes. Thankfully, for those wanting to paddle, the shoreline stretch along **East Ocean Boulevard** lies separate from the commercial district. The street is relatively easy to navigate and offers a decent amount of free parking.

East Ocean Boulevard follows a peninsula that runs between **Alamitos Bay** and the breakwater. Obviously a peninsula has water on both sides, and consequently there are two opportunities for paddling: the breakwater, on the ocean side of the peninsula, and Alamitos Bay, on the inland side. The breakwater constitutes a large swath of ocean protected by the network of jetties that form the Port

Belmont Shore

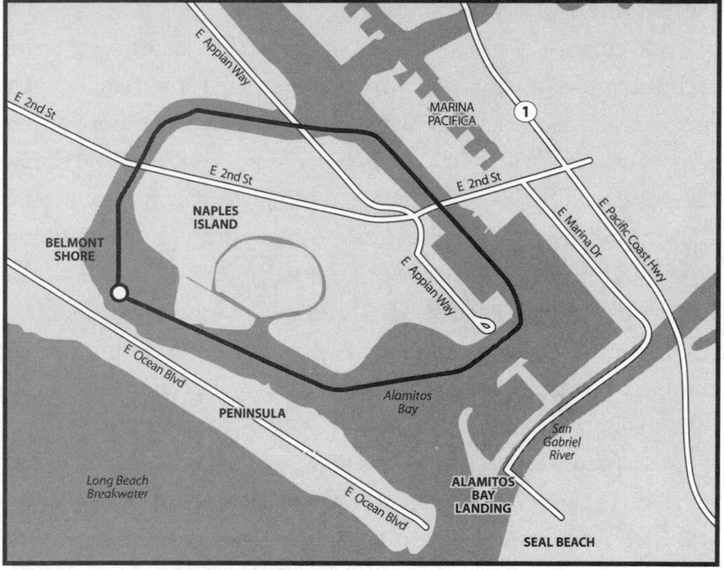

of Long Beach. The *Queen Mary* is docked at the west end of this reach. The jetties generally block all incoming surf, and the beach has become a popular flat-water spot for local kiteboarders. Alamitos Bay consists of several narrow channels and inlets, all lined with beachfront real estate and docked pleasure boats. The bay is popular with just about every form of human-powered craft: kayaks, pedal boats, one-design windsurfers, Venice-style gondolas, open-water swimmers, and SUP boards.

WHERE TO PADDLE Summer crowds often flock to both of these areas, but for paddling I recommend avoiding the breakwater and heading to the bay. The first reason is obvious: It's a much shorter walk to the water on the bay side. The wide beach in front of the breakwater means a long trek with board in hand. The breakwater is also much windier than the bay, hence its popularity with kiteboarders, and its shoreline is famous for stingrays (I've been stung there on two different occasions). And when it comes to scenery, the breakwater is mostly big, ugly, and industrial.

In contrast, Alamitos Bay has a certain charm: bridges, boats, and plenty of attractive shorefront properties. It's a friendly destination where locals and tourists gather to enjoy some time on the water. On calm days, the 1.8-mile course around **Naples Island** should take most paddlers 30–45 minutes to complete. It's a pleasant route, allowing for plenty of sights and people-watching. One Saturday a year, on the weekend nearest St. Patrick's Day, the course is also the site of the **Adler Paddler**—a race/family paddle event/fundraiser that's free and open to everyone (see page 100 for more information). It's a worthwhile cause to support, as well a fun event for paddlers of all ability levels.

The route around Naples Island is simple and easy to follow. Start at the strand just below **Bay Shore Avenue.** The beach is wide and spacious here, and launching couldn't be easier. Heading clockwise, paddle toward the **Second Street Bridge.** Continue under the bridge, following the relatively narrow channel between homes and docks that leads to the **Appian Way Bridge.** Veer right into the wider channel just east of **Marine Stadium,** and then cross again under the Second Street Bridge. At this point, the course passes a large network of boat docks, heading in the direction of Seal Beach and the jetty for the San Gabriel River, which separates Alamitos Bay from Seal Beach (and Los Angeles County from Orange County).

Turn right at the **Alamitos Bay Marina Center**—there is no other way to turn—and into the mouth of Alamitos Bay, continuing away from Seal Beach. This stretch can be windy, particularly on summer afternoons when the sea breezes pick up. If this is the case, try to paddle toward the westward shore, finding some protected waters along the leeward side of the peninsula. Here, a series of sandy beaches also offers opportunities to stop and rest. (For most this won't be a difficult paddle, but the wind can be a factor.) Complete the loop by following the channel between the peninsula and Naples Island back to the launch point.

Please note that the wind can be strong here. The presence of kiteboarders inside the breakwater generally indicates a strong headwind on the last leg of the route. In this case, paddlers have two options: The first is to follow the course counterclockwise; there will still be a headwind on the backside of the loop, but it shouldn't be as strong as the wind that blows across the mouth of Alamitos Bay. The other option is to forgo the loop around Naples Island and instead paddle the canals inside of Naples Island. This may be a quaint option even on nonwindy days—a shorter tour that is favored by for-hire gondoliers as well as many paddlers. For this option, simply launch at the aforementioned beach and paddle straight across the channel to Naples Island. The closest entrance to the canals is near **Naples Elementary School.** Veer right at the school and then left to navigate into the interior of the island. The narrow canals form a loop inside the shores of the island.

DIRECTIONS AND PARKING From Pacific Coast Highway, follow Second Street west for 1.1 miles, then turn left on Bay Shore Avenue. Continue along the water, first on Bayshore and then on 54th Place, until you reach East Ocean Boulevard. Turn left on East Ocean; the launch is on the left-hand side.

Note: Bay Shore Avenue may be closed to traffic in the summer months, in which case a slight detour is necessary: Proceed to the first stop light at Santa Ana Avenue, turn left, and then follow the street until it ends at East Ocean Boulevard.

Free street parking is available on both sides of East Ocean Boulevard; there is also a narrow lot adjacent to the bay with metered parking spots.

CONDITIONS AND HAZARDS The breakwater is famous for stingrays, but the bay is safe, calm, and easily accessed. Again, though, winds can be strong here: Afternoon sea breezes push around Palos Verdes and accelerate through the corridor between Long Beach and Huntington Beach. During the summer months, conditions will be more favorable in the morning.

RENTALS On the beach, adjacent to the launch area, **Standup Rentals** (5411 E. Ocean Blvd.; 562-434-0999, **standuprentals.net**) offers board-storage facilities and rentals. From April to October, they're open every day from 9 a.m. to sunset; in the winter, they're open on most weekends, depending on weather conditions. Basic rentals are $25 per hour, but there are membership discounts and early-bird specials.

ADLER PADDLER Named in memory of local surfer, board shaper, and stand-up paddler Steve Adler, this SUP race began in 2012 as a fundraiser for The John Ritter Foundation for Aortic Health (**johnritter foundation.org**). The goal of the event is to bring the paddling community together for a morning of fun and exercise while raising money and awareness for thoracic aortic dissection—a genetic heart defect that killed both Steve Adler and John Ritter (and, it should be noted, the author's father). Registration is free, but proceeds are raised through board rentals, T-shirt sales, and raffle sales (see **paddlewith purpose.wordpress.com** for raffle items). Participants who don't have an SUP board may arrive early and rent a board as a donation to the cause. The event consists of two race classes and a family-friendly paddle around the course for nonracers. Expert-level racers make two laps around the course; noncompetitors launch behind the racers, so everyone is on the water at once.

Cabrillo Beach

San Pedro (Los Angeles)

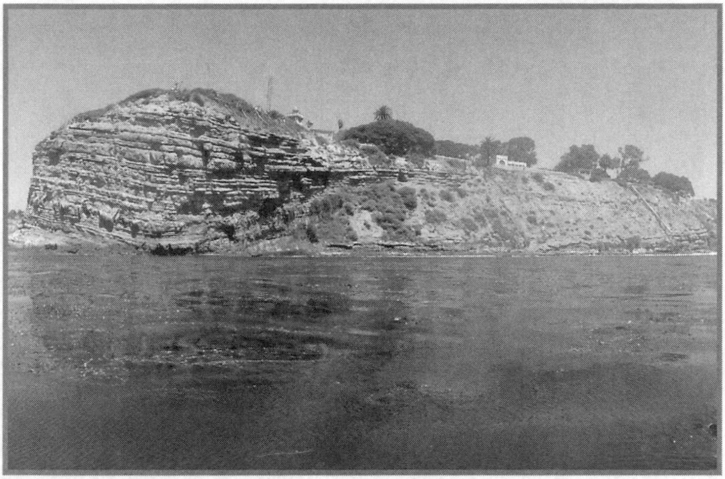

Kelp beds outside of Point Fermin

OVERVIEW Juan Rodríguez Cabrillo, a Portuguese explorer, discovered San Pedro Bay in 1542. At the time, the inlet was merely a shallow mudflat, unable to support a wharf, let alone harbor ships. But as Los Angeles grew in size and stature, so did its need for a functioning port. In 1871, spurred by the completion of a railroad line, the bay was dredged and construction of the Port of Los Angeles soon followed. These days, the former mudflat is one of the busiest shipping centers in the world.

Cabrillo Beach lies at the western edge of the massive port, a narrow haven of sand and rock jetties between the leeward edge of **Palos Verdes** and the sprawling complex of **Los Angeles Harbor.** Stand on the beach here and look east, and it's hard not to be awestruck by the size and the density of the harbor's construction. The **Vincent Thomas Bridge** towers over a vast collection of docks and cranes and impossibly large ships. To the west are the equally vast Pacific Ocean and, more specifically, the channel between **Point Fermin** and **Catalina Island.** (Although I'm not recommending a paddle to Catalina, Cabrillo Beach is one of the closest points on the mainland to the island.)

WHERE TO PADDLE For water access, the best parking at Cabrillo is in the narrow lot between the outer beach and the harbor jetty. Here, one is equally close to the harbor and the open ocean. Paddling in the bay might be an option for some—it's really only recommended for beginners—but most SUPers will want to head out into the ocean. Unless there is a large groundswell, the waves at Cabrillo are fairly tame and break close to shore. If the shore break near the jetty looks daunting, try launching at the western edge of the beach, closer to the cliffs and tidepools.

Paddle west from the beach, first parallel to the long crescent of sand and then around the cliffs of Point Fermin. Within minutes, you'll be removed from the busy world of the port, entering the quieter waters off the Palos Verdes Peninsula. Of course, this is still San Pedro, so don't expect to see the manicured landscapes of Palos Verdes proper. The picture-perfect estates and Donald Trump's golf course are still several miles to the north. Near Point Fermin, the cliffs are dotted with chain-link fences, graffiti-covered walls, and unexpected bursts of flora. (I spied one cliffside lot with a collection of

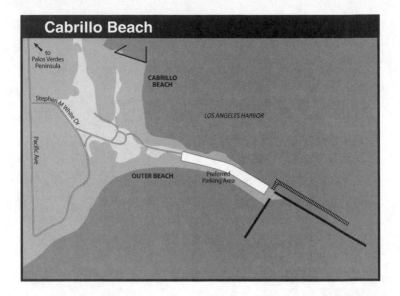

stalky century cacti, all listing or toppled from exposure to the wind.) This area is also home to the **Sunken City of San Pedro,** a clifftop sinkhole that is officially off-limits but unofficially an offbeat local attraction that seems to appeal to loitering teenagers and a peculiar subset of adventure tourists. Far below, on the water, the scenery is much more typical—striated cliffs and rocky shoals, thriving kelp beds, and a host of marine life.

Continuing west, then northwest, it's roughly a 2-mile paddle to **Royal Palms State Beach.** The course will take you around to the windward side of Point Fermin and then along another cliff-lined strand. A series of scallop-shaped reefs marks narrow **White Point,** and just beyond that lies Royal Palms—easily recognized by its signature trees. Because of the density of reefs and rocks near White Point, landing is difficult here, and therefore not recommended. There is one pebbly cove at the north end of the park and beach, but most paddlers will do better to enjoy the view from the water. Remaining offshore has its attractions; the reefs of White Point are also popular with divers—giant crabs, bat rays, and harmless leopard sharks are commonly seen in these waters.

Overall, this route is quite satisfying. It's hard to believe that such a scenic coastline lies so close to a massive shipping hub. When paddling close to the cliffs, one has the impression of being close to a remote, unpopulated shore—not an experience typically found near L.A. Harbor.

The day I made the trip, the water was remarkably clear; however, there was a fairly substantial headwind. Cabrillo Beach is a popular windsurfing spot, so afternoon winds are prevalent here and often quite strong. In the summer months, particularly when the temperatures soar inland, expect to encounter a steady flow of thermal winds pushing around Point Fermin. Try to make this paddle in the morning: Because of the westward exposure of the point, the sea breezes can arrive relatively early, often starting around noon and then remaining for much of the day. If there is a headwind, the trip to Royal Palms will require some vigorous effort, but because of the

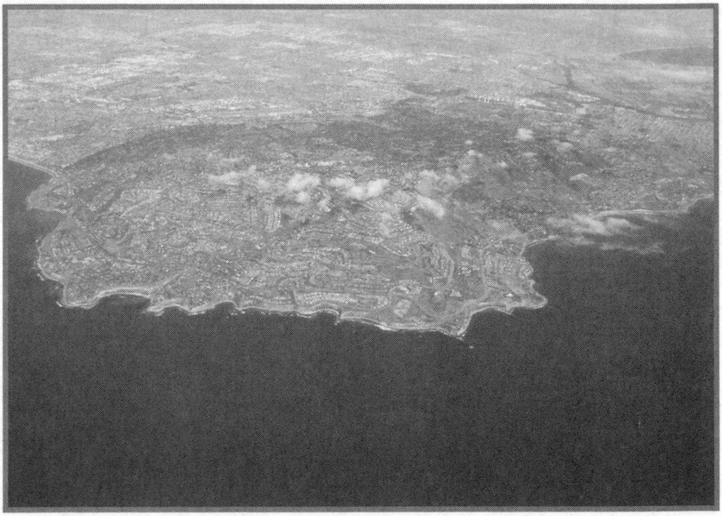

Clifftop view of the Palos Verdes Peninsula

kelp barrier, these waters aren't as choppy as they could be—paddling into the stiff headwind was difficult, but not prohibitively difficult. Then, of course, the return trip was all downwind . . . a breeze.

Perhaps the ultimate attraction of Cabrillo is convenience. For many Southland residents, this launch offers the most direct access to the waters of the Palos Verdes Peninsula. The beach feels a bit industrial, even dirty, but the surrounding area is definitely worth exploring. It may be possible to launch at Royal Palms State Beach, but the rocky shore makes this prospect less appealing. The sandy shore at Cabrillo is ideal for hauling boards in and out of the water.

For beginners, there is also the bay side of Cabrillo. Here you'll find a long sandy beach for launching and calmer (boat-free) water to paddle through. The downside to the bay is the water quality—often rated as some of the dirtiest in Los Angeles—and the industrial setting. So for most paddlers, I recommend heading out into the ocean.

DIRECTIONS AND PARKING Take I-110 west toward San Pedro. When the freeway ends, exit left onto North Gaffey Street. Follow

North Gaffey for 1.5 miles, then turn left onto West 22nd Street. At the bottom of the hill, turn right onto South Pacific Avenue, then turn left on Stephen M. White Drive, heading into the beach park. Past the entrance gate, stay to the right and then follow the road out to the parking lot near the jetty. Ample parking is available most days, but the lot may fill on summer weekends. Parking runs $1 per hour and up to $9 per day.

CONDITIONS AND HAZARDS The beach is sandy and the launch friendly, but there can be a shore break. On most days, a little timing is all that's required to get out through the surf. Some paddlers may want to walk to the western end of the beach, where the break is smaller. Waves also break over a few rocky shoals to the west of the beach, but these are both easy to spot and easy to avoid.

Watch out for broken glass in the parking lot, and be aware of the possibility of car theft. Some local windsurfers have complained about break-ins on weekends, although I don't think they're that common.

Local windsurfers sometimes refer to Cabrillo as "Hurricane Gulch." The nickname is definitely an exaggeration, but take heed—wind can be a factor here. Start paddling early in the day, and always paddle west (windward) first.

LOCAL BURRITO Burrito Factory, about five blocks from the beach on Pacific Avenue, has a menu full of burritos: 20 separate options, each served with a side salad and chips. Per usual, I tried the chile relleno burrito; it was satisfying but not memorable—more like a diced-green-chile burrito with beans. You can eat in or get your food to go, but if you order takeout and plan to eat in your car, be prepared for a mess. My burrito was definitely a fork-and-knife experience, exploding all over the place. Word on the street is that this place was better before it changed ownership. The location is definitely convenient to Cabrillo Beach, but I wouldn't drive out of my way to eat here. (1902 S. Pacific Ave.; 310-547-9001, **burritofactorysp.com.**)

ABALONE COVE **Palos Verdes**

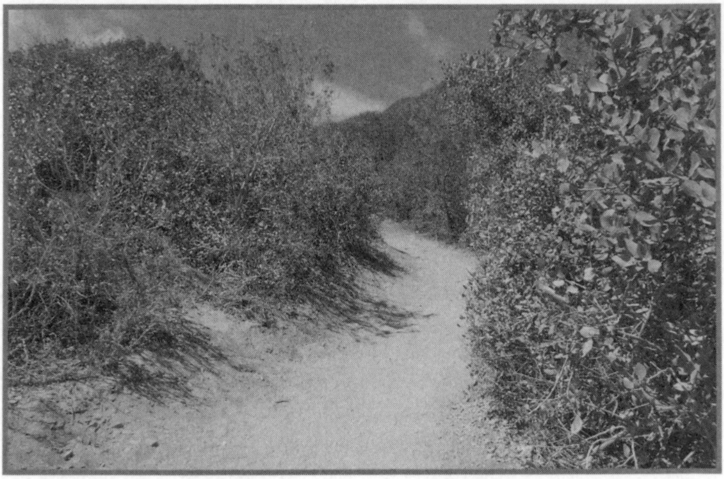

The hiking trail down to Abalone Cove

OVERVIEW It's hard to believe Palos Verdes is even part of greater Los Angeles. The cliff-lined peninsula, with its remote, rocky beaches and rolling hillsides, seems like it should be located somewhere between Big Sur and Monterey. Unlike other coastal areas in Southern California, the peninsula has not been completely blotted out by development. Many of the hillsides have been spared the work of graders, and many of the coastal cliffs are still unblemished. A drive around Palos Verdes is quite a treat, with plenty of unobstructed views of the rolling hills and the dramatic coastline.

Because of the cliffs, the beaches on the peninsula are not as easily reached as those in other parts of Los Angeles, thus they are remarkably uncrowded. They are also remarkably scenic. Abalone Cove is no exception: It's a beautiful beach that requires a bit of effort to get to. For the paddleboarder, this will mean carrying one's board down a dirt path, then launching along a rock-strewn beach. On the day I paddled at Abalone, I was the only SUPer on the water, and for all I know, I may have been the only paddler there the entire week.

Parking for the cove is located directly off **Palos Verdes Drive.** (At this writing, the main lot is being reconstructed and should

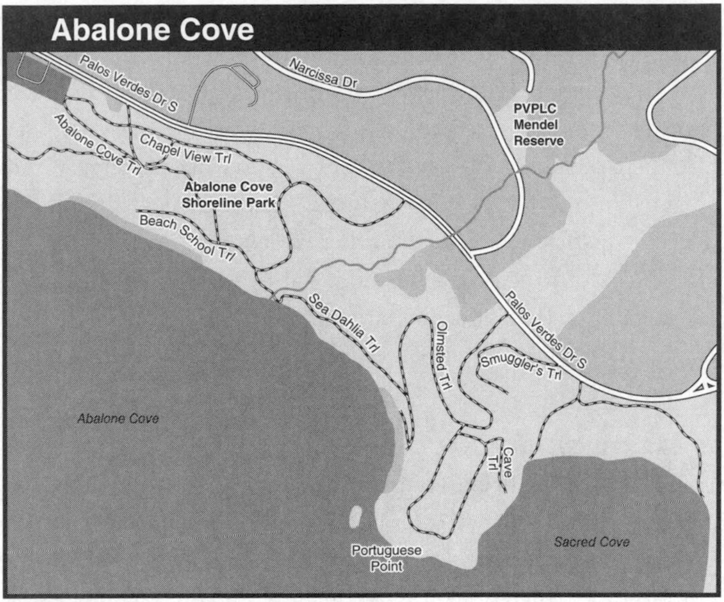

be finished, along with a newly designed clifftop park, by summer 2015.) When I pulled in, the attendant told me it was a 30-minute walk to the beach. After discussing the condition of the trail, he offered to give me my parking money back if it was too difficult to heft my board all the way to the beach. It wasn't. With my board in a carrying strap, the 10- to 15-minute walk (maybe 10 minutes for the trip down and 15 minutes for the trip back up) seemed only mildly strenuous. The path is a well-maintained dirt trail, not too steep and wide enough to navigate while packing an SUP board.

At the bottom of the hill, near a lifeguard facility, the trail splits to the north and the south. I took the south option, and the slightly longer walk, because I wanted to paddle in that direction. I'm not sure if this was the best decision; the beach north of the lifeguard building appeared to be somewhat friendlier for launching.

The beach at Abalone Cove is covered with biscuit-sized stones. The shoreline is also steeply angled, so getting in and (particularly) out of the water can be a bit tricky. Regarding my earlier statement, the beach north of the lifeguard station seemed less steep, so climbing out of the water there may be less difficult. However, the stones are everywhere, so for those with sensitive feet, I would recommend wearing booties. Another option is to wear shoes into the water, then take them off and attach them to your person while paddling. (Crocs are good for this because they're lightweight, they float, and they're ugly enough that no one ever minds dunking them in salt water.)

Now for the good part: Paddling at Abalone Cove is an amazing experience. Below the dramatic cliffs is a perfectly beautiful seascape—hidden beaches and craggy points lined with reefs, tidepools, and sea caves.

WHERE TO PADDLE From the launch, I opted to paddle south around **Portuguese Point,** along the protected waters of **Sacred Cove,** and then outside the narrower outcropping of **Inspiration Point.** The pristine sandy beach of Sacred Cove, protected by the twin promontories of Portuguese Point and Inspiration Point and accessible only by water or a steep hiking trail, seemed like a coastal Shangri-La—too beautiful and too remote to be part of L.A. County (I know I've said this before, but it's worth repeating). The water in the cove was clear and aquamarine from the reflection of sunlight off the smooth, sandy seabed. The beach appeared perfectly inviting and absolutely empty.

At the north end, just to the lee of Portuguese Point, a sea cave flushes through to Abalone Cove. This is not a cave for paddling or swimming, but the sight of the hydraulics—waves funneling through the narrow gap in the cliff—was a highlight of the trip.

Working my way back around Portuguese Point, I was forced to endure a bit of current and headwind, but once inside Abalone Cove, the paddling was relatively easy. The windward side of the point has a couple of rocky channels and, closer to the cliffs, a network of tidepools. It's possible to paddle near the pools, but closer inspection (for those wanting to investigate the minutiae of the marine life) requires a hike out to the point.

Overall, I was quite impressed with the location and the paddle. For those wanting to make the trip, I advise going early—before the wind comes up—and allowing enough paddling time to make the trip worthwhile. Obviously, this paddle won't be for everyone. For those wanting to experience the Palos Verdes Peninsula without the board portage, launching at **Cabrillo Beach** or **RAT Beach** near Redondo will be preferable (see previous and following profiles).

DIRECTIONS AND PARKING From the Long Beach area, take I-710 South and exit at Pico Avenue. Turn right onto Pico, then merge onto CA 47, heading over the Vincent Thomas Bridge to San Pedro. After 4.8 miles, take the Gaffey Street exit and head toward San Pedro (Gaffey becomes Summerland Avenue). Head straight for 1 mile, then turn left on Western Avenue and continue for 2 miles. Turn right onto 25th Street, which after a mile becomes Palos Verdes Drive. Continue along the divided road for another 2.5 miles, looking for the signs to Abalone Cove. Just past the cove, make a U-turn at Archery Range Road, then head back to the parking lot. Parking is $5.

CONDITIONS AND HAZARDS This is a remote and inaccessible stretch of coastline. Lifeguards are stationed at Abalone Cove, but I doubt they'd be able to assist those paddling outside of the sight lines of the cove. As always, be aware of your paddling ability and your experience level.

The beach here is completely covered in rocks, making for difficult footing. Climbing out of the water over the loose stones with a board in hand can be a bit tricky. Booties are recommended for the tenderfooted.

Because of its westward protrusion and tall cliffs, Palos Verdes has fairly focused sea breezes, as well as slightly cooler water temperatures due to upwelling. In the summer, expect winds to pick up in the afternoon. In the winter months, this beach may be prone to large surf.

FACILITIES There are picnic benches and restrooms at the top of the cliff.

RAT Beach

Redondo Beach

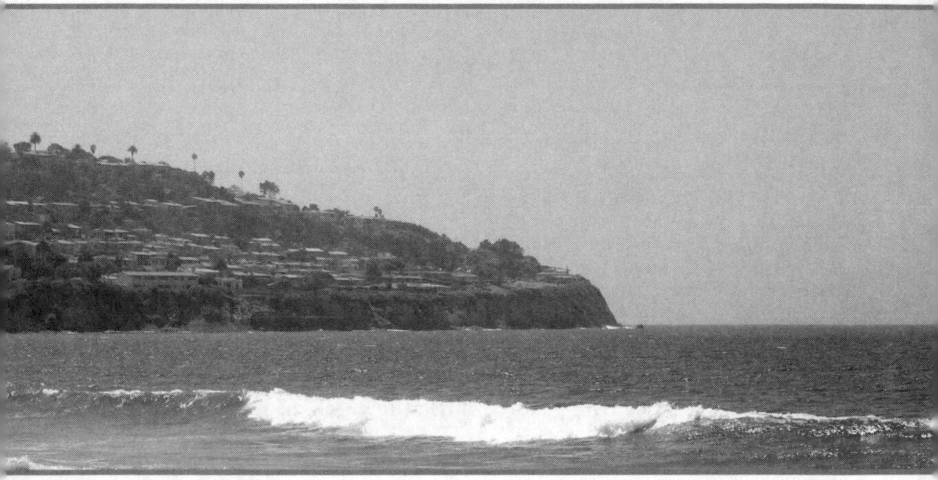

View from RAT Beach toward the cliffs of the Palos Verdes Peninsula

OVERVIEW *RAT* is a local acronym for "Right After Torrance." The moniker refers to the southernmost strand of the South Bay, an open length of sand that stretches down to the cliffs of Palos Verdes. The wide city beach is popular with local beachgoers; out in the water, one typically finds small packs of surfers and bodyboarders spread across numerous sections of beach break. At least during the summer, RAT is known for small surf and relatively uncrowded conditions. Because of the amount of space and the lack of a competitive vibe (beginner surfers frequent this beach), RAT is also popular with a crew of stand-up surfers. A multitude of peaks break along this beach—some better than others—but it's often possible to stake out a wave of one's own.

For those who prefer to paddle outside the surf, RAT Beach is an excellent starting point to access scenic Palos Verdes. It's only about a 10- to 15-minute paddle to the northern edge of the peninsula and roughly a 45-minute paddle to the majestic cliffs at **Flat Rock Point.** Coursing through these waters provides an excellent opportunity to view marine life and to take in panoramic views of the peninsula, the South Bay, and downtown Los Angeles.

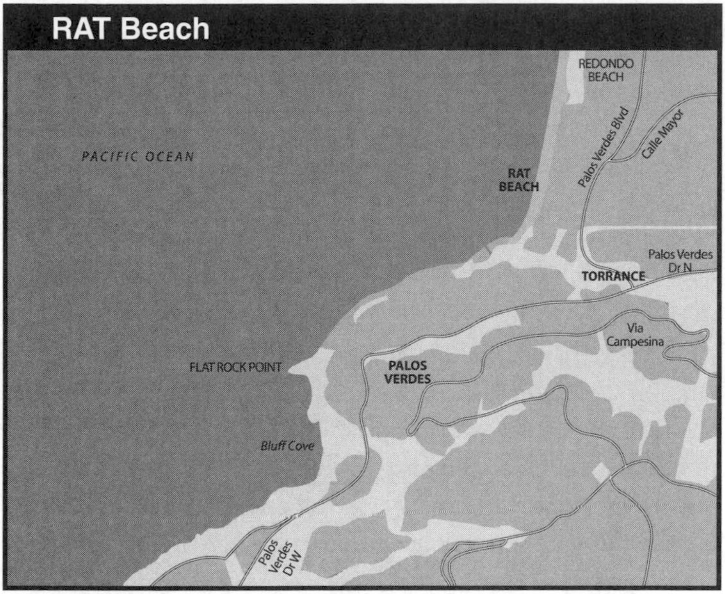

WHERE TO PADDLE To reach the launch at RAT Beach, park at the south end of the city lot off Paseo de la Playa (you'll probably see other vehicles with SUP boards), pay at the kiosk, and then walk down the short sandy path to the beach. A concrete path also leads to the beach, but the sand route is more direct. The beach offers plenty of space to launch boards, and for the most part, the crowds seem to thin as one heads farther south.

The paddle along RAT Beach is relatively unremarkable, but upon reaching the rocky edge of the peninsula, there is much more to see. On the day I paddled this stretch, I saw a few intrepid divers accessing the isolated shore via a steep rope-lined trail. I also saw several fishermen scrambling over rocks, racing against the incoming tide. The coast here is essentially a long series of reefs, many of them tucked inside thriving kelp beds. It's easy to see the beach's appeal for divers and fishermen.

As you head out to the point, the cliffs grow taller and steeper. At Flat Rock Point, the bluff appeared to be 300–400 feet above sea level. Beyond the point is **Bluff Cove** (also called **PV Cove**), a rocky inlet where yellow-clay cliffs rise above emerald-green water. A trail leads down to the cove, and when the surf is good, the break tends to be a popular longboarding spot. In the winter, there can be substantial surf at PV Cove, enticing some South Bay stand-up surfers to make the paddle out here (probably easier than carrying boards down the trail). But the surfing area tends to be crowded and not nearly as friendly as RAT Beach—although PV Cove is a much better wave when it breaks. (It seems there's often a trade-off between wave quality and crowds.)

For those not concerned about waves, there is plenty to see here. Perhaps one of the cherished aspects of stand-up paddling is the ability to explore new, out-of-the-way places, and this paddle seems to meet that criterion. From the point, there are nice views of the South Bay, the nearby cove, and the collection of reefs immediately outside the point. I recommend this paddle for anyone wanting to explore a bit of nature and perhaps find a bit of solitude. The launch is friendly, and the paddle out to the point is not particularly difficult. One small challenge may be dealing with a bit of wave refraction from the cliffs. For those feeling unstable on their boards, paddling farther away from the rocky shoreline will make for easier going.

As I mentioned earlier, the surf tends to be small at RAT Beach; the exception will be during winter west and northwest swells. In these conditions, particularly when the swell is more than 4 feet, the cliffs south of RAT Beach create a long point break. Known as **Haggerty's,** the wave is often crowded with an aggressive crew of surfers. If the point is breaking, paddlers may want to take a bit of caution and follow a route away from the cliffs through deeper water.

DIRECTIONS AND PARKING If you don't live in the South Bay, getting here always seems difficult. The closest freeway, I-405, runs several miles inland from the coast, but perhaps that's what keeps these beaches from being overrun with tourists. From Pacific Coast Highway, head south on Palos Verdes Boulevard for 0.8 mile. Turn right on Calle Miramar, then immediately left on Via Riviera. After

0.1 mile, turn right onto Paseo de la Playa; the parking lot will be immediately on the left. After entering, park at the far south end of the lot and look for the sandy trail to the beach. Parking costs $5 per day in summer and $3 per day in the off-season.

CONDITIONS AND HAZARDS The beach is sandy and wide open, and the surf is often smaller and more forgiving than other area beaches. In winter, the point (Haggerty's) can produce large, fast waves, attracting enthusiastic crowds of surfers. Otherwise, the vibe is pretty laid-back and the surf uncrowded.

As with every ocean beach, wind can be an issue, but RAT Beach should typically be less windy than Cabrillo Beach or Abalone Cove.

LOCAL BURRITO El Burrito Jr. (919 S. Pacific Coast Highway.; 310-316-5058) is an institution in Redondo Beach. It's the Mexican-food experience so many Californians were raised on—fast, inexpensive, and richly comforting. There's no inside seating here; all orders are taken at the window at the front of the A-frame building. Expect a crowd during lunch and dinner. Locals may argue about who has the best burrito in Redondo, but El Burrito Jr. has great street visibility and a long-standing reputation for ample portions and reasonable prices.

KING HARBOR **Redondo Beach**

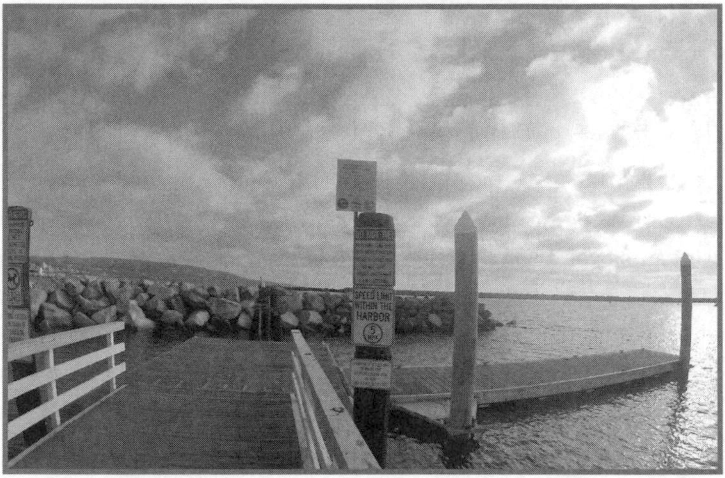

The public dock at King Harbor

OVERVIEW Stand-up paddling has definitely taken hold in the South Bay. And why not? It's a great place to paddle. Here, one finds long stretches of sandy beach, plenty of open water, and fairly easy coastal access (particularly when compared with cliff-lined Palos Verdes and fenced-off Malibu). From Torrance to Redondo, and between the piers at Hermosa Beach and Manhattan Beach, stand-up paddlers are a common sight—cruising, training, and riding waves.

Of course, the open ocean isn't for everyone, particularly when afternoon sea breezes chop up the water surface. So, for consistent flat-water paddling in the South Bay, King Harbor is an ideal location. The marina, which is just north of the Redondo Beach pier, has a tall, protective jetty that provides a barrier against those afternoon sea breezes. (The jetty runs almost directly north–south, so it works well as a buffer against west winds). On the leeward side of the jetty, the water tends to remain smooth even when the ocean is filled with whitecaps. This is a perfect spot for beginner paddlers and for anyone who prefers their sunset paddle to be relaxing rather than vigorous. Moreover, for those who desire a diversity of conditions, it's only a short paddle from the protected launch to the ocean beyond the breakwater.

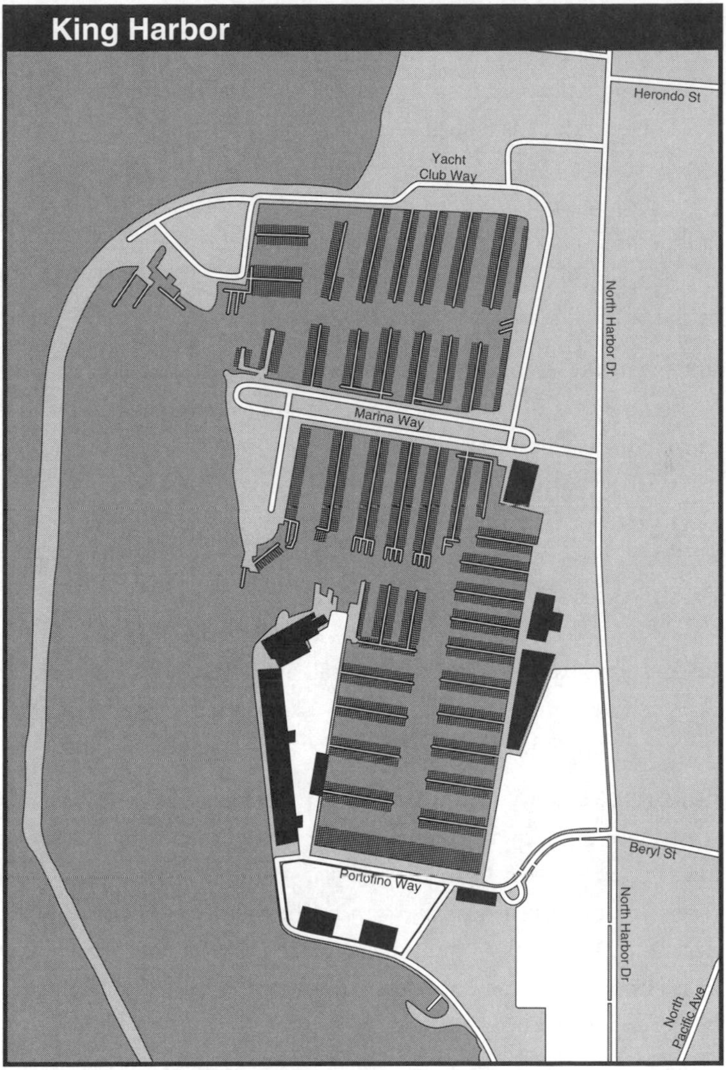

Besides SUPers, an active group of outrigger paddlers plies the waters of King Harbor. Every February, the local club puts on the **Lanakila Carpet Beach Classic** (see page 117 for more information).

WHERE TO PADDLE Although there are plenty of private docks to launch from, there's really only one public launch in King Harbor—a short, no-frills dock just behind **Ruby's Restaurant** on North Harbor Drive. Parking is plentiful in the adjacent public lot (payment is required), and a flat concrete path leads to the water. From the public dock, it's just a quick paddle out into the main channel of the harbor, and perhaps only a 5-minute paddle out into the open water. This is the biggest advantage of paddling King Harbor—going from the car to the water in a matter of minutes.

DIRECTIONS AND PARKING From Pacific Coast Highway in Redondo Beach, head west on Torrance Boulevard, then take the second right on South Catalina Avenue. Continue 0.5 mile, then turn left on Beryl Street. Head down the slight grade, then turn left at North Harbor Drive. The parking-lot entrance will be on the right-hand side. Park to the south of Ruby's Restaurant (245 N. Harbor Drive), as close to the water as possible.

To get to the bay access, follow the concrete path past On the Rocks sports bar and look for the small public dock (it's just inside a short, curved jetty). Parking runs $1–$2 per hour, depending on the season. Take a ticket at the gate and pay as you exit.

CONDITIONS AND HAZARDS Safe and sane. Be a little cautious when heading out past the breakwater—the ocean current may be much stronger than in the bay, and if you get pushed downwind, there isn't much beach to land at near the pier. Note that the public dock also has a small amount of current. Be careful not to leave your board unmanned (and untethered) in the water before launching, or it may end up washing into the nearby rocks.

RENTALS **Tarsan Stand-Up Paddle Boarding** (831 N. Harbor Drive; 310-798-2200, **tarsanstandup.com**), about a mile north of the public dock and just south of the power plant on North Harbor, offers rentals, lessons, and fun group-paddle events. Tarsan also has its own private access to the harbor and offers free parking for customers, so

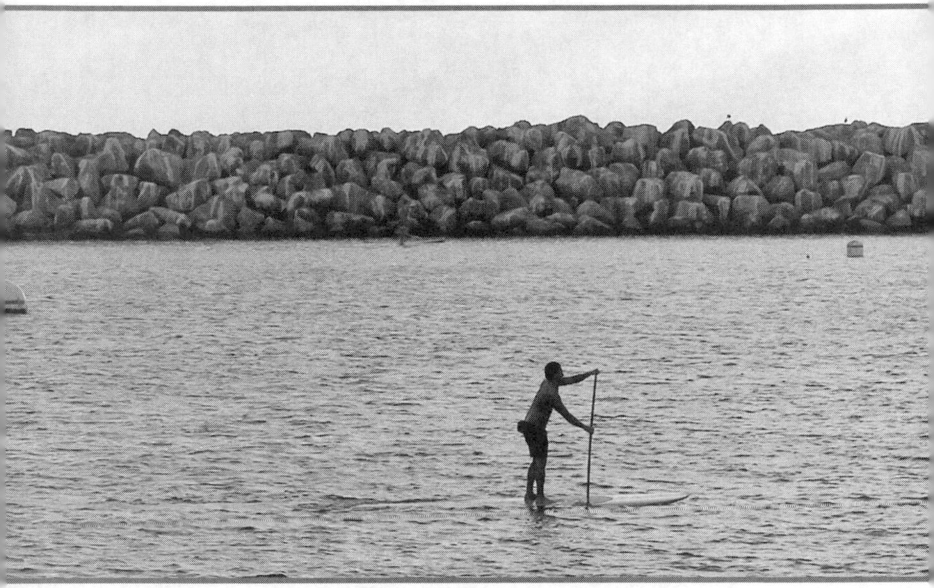

A lone paddler courses through King Harbor.

it's an easy and convenient option for those new to the sport. (Tarsan also has a shop in Hermosa Beach, but only the Redondo location has direct water access.)

LANAKILA CARPET BEACH CLASSIC Although this race started as an event exclusively for outrigger canoeists, it has since become quite popular with stand-up paddlers. The 5-mile short course begins in the harbor, makes a loop outside the pier, and then finishes back inside the harbor. Visit **lanakila.com** for more information, or check with the folks at Tarsan Stand-Up Paddle Boarding.

MARINA DEL REY **Los Angeles**

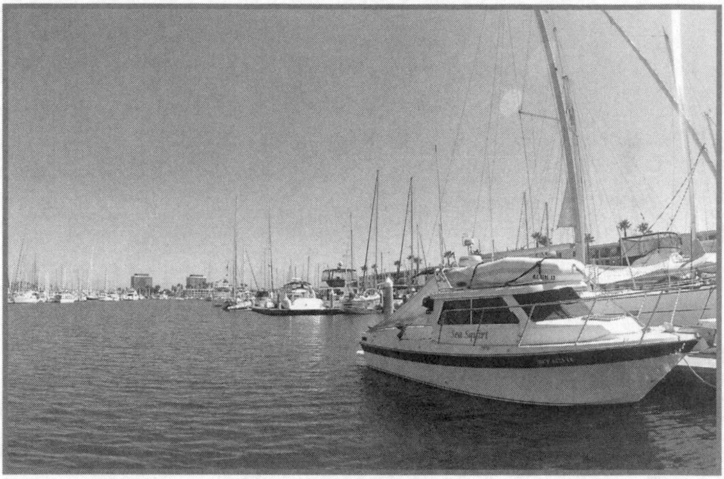

Heading out Basin D among a multitude of masts

OVERVIEW In 1962, the SS *Minnow* pulled out of these waters, ready to embark on its fateful trip. Its unintended destination: a fictional uncharted island that spawned three seasons of television comedy and a catchy theme song.

Marina Del Rey was the backdrop for *Gilligan's Island*'s opening credits, and the harbor's associations with movie stars and millionaires haven't changed much in 50 years. When I paddled here on a sunny September weekday, there were plenty of yachts on the water, and although I didn't see any movie stars, I did see a film crew shooting outside, taking advantage of the clear skies and Kodachrome-blue water.

The marina, which happens to be the largest man-made harbor in the world, lies just west of the LAX flight pattern. More than 6,000 boats find safe haven here, docked in a series of basins and surrounded by high-rise hotels and condominiums. It's a big space for paddling, and although most of the docks are private, there is public parking and public access at **Mother's Beach.**

WHERE TO PADDLE Mother's Beach might have the most user-friendly paddling launch in Los Angeles. It's only a short walk from

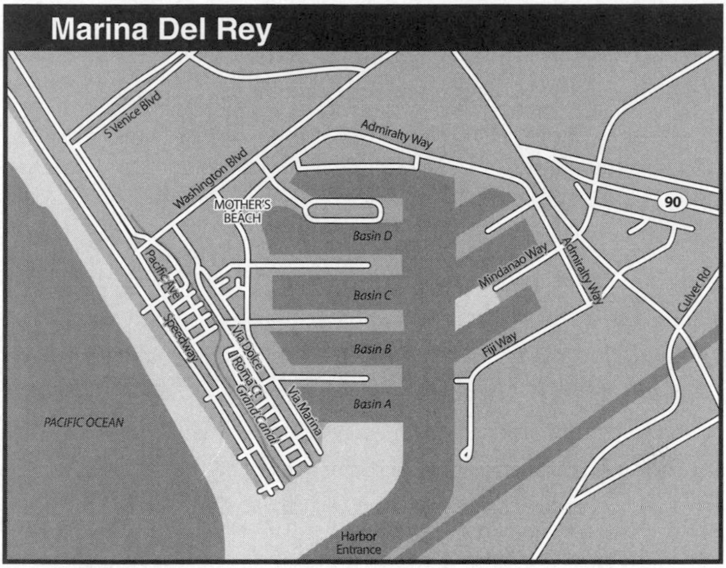

the parking area to a concrete walkway that heads directly into the bay. The beach also has shaded picnic tables and volleyball nets. It's the perfect place for group parties and group paddling sessions. When I was here, several novice paddlers were testing the calm waters near the launch. If you want to get someone out on the water, perhaps someone who's afraid of waves and the open ocean or just water in general, this is the place to take them. For confident paddlers, there is ample acreage for longer paddles.

And there is plenty to see—6,000 boats for one. Among other things, Marina Del Rey is famous for its upscale waterfront real estate. Paddling here is almost like window-shopping—peeking into a world of affluence. That's not to say it isn't friendly: Boats travel slowly and wake-free in the harbor, people wave, and even the seals seem happy.

From Mother's Beach, it's roughly a 40-minute paddle to the harbor entrance (depending on wind). The directions are simple—just leave the beach and head out Basin D toward the main channel of the harbor. Turn right at the channel and keep paddling south toward the main jetty.

As you head out of the harbor, you're bound to see a few planes leaving from LAX, and just beyond the jetty are the cliff-lined **Ballona Wetlands.** However, the majority of the scenery at Marina Del Rey is nautical. The docks play host to a seemingly limitless collection of pleasure craft. If you even have a casual interest in boating, you'll find plenty here to pique your curiosity.

Near the harbor entrance there tends to be a bit more wind and chop. It's still protected, but headwinds tend to push straight up the mouth of the jetty. The trip home should be mostly downwind, although you might encounter a headwind after making the final turn to Mother's Beach. Be careful on your way back—the basins look deceptively similar, and you may be unsure where to turn. When returning from the harbor mouth, just take the fourth basin on the left and you should end up where you started.

DIRECTIONS AND PARKING From I-405, take the Marina Freeway (CA 90) west toward Marina Del Rey. After 2.8 miles, turn left on Mindanao Way. After crossing Lincoln Boulevard (CA 1), make the first right onto Admiralty Way. Continue for 1.3 miles, then, just past the Jamaica Bay Inn, make a left turn into the parking lot at Mother's Beach. Find a space and then pay at the machine. Rates are $1–$1.50 per hour, depending on the season.

CONDITIONS AND HAZARDS Easy and stress-free. I didn't see any notable hazards, but always pay attention. During my paddle, after becoming completely awestruck while looking up at a massive sailboat, I managed to clumsily topple into the water. (In my defense, it was the tallest sailboat in the world—a 90-meter mast!)

FACILITIES Restrooms, shaded picnic tables, and volleyball courts are all nearby. A concrete pathway to the water makes launching a snap.

RENTALS AND LESSONS **Pro SUP Shop** (4175 Admiralty Way; 310-945-8350, **prosupshop.com**) is located in the southwest corner of the Jamaica Bay Inn parking lot, adjacent to Mother's Beach. They offer rentals, lessons, and guided SUP cruises.

Malibu Pier and Escondido Beach

Malibu

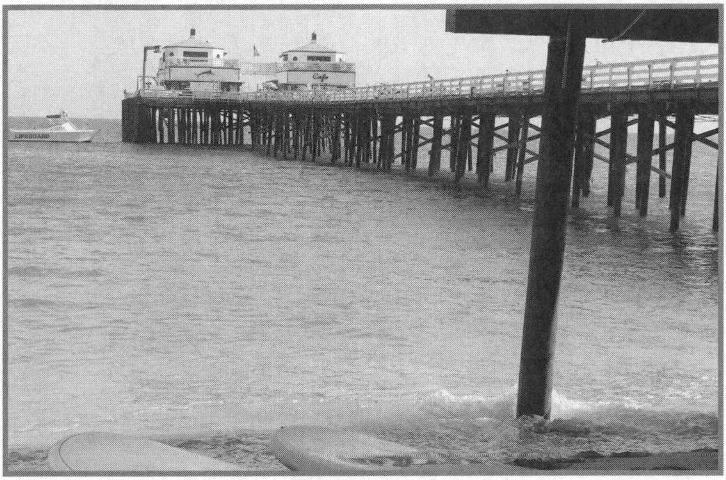

The narrow launch spot just south of the Malibu Pier

OVERVIEW TWENTY-SEVEN MILES OF SCENIC BEAUTY—that's what the highway signs herald near Malibu's city limits. And it's a claim that's pretty difficult to argue with. Malibu, or "The Bu" as locals call it, is a spectacular place—a long, narrow stretch of coastline tucked beneath the steep rise of the Santa Monica Mountains.

Malibu has plenty of beautiful beaches, but they aren't always easy to access. Much of the Malibu coast is lined with expensive homes, and many of the homeowners are less than amenable to allowing public access. Thankfully, for those without beachfront homes, several state and city parks lie along this stretch of coast, as well as a few public easements. For those wanting more information on the subject, the **Los Angeles Urban Rangers** publish a guide to Malibu's public beaches (see page 125). Note, however, that not all of the guide's access points are ideal for SUP boards—some require negotiating narrow staircases or steep trails.

WHERE TO PADDLE Ground zero in Malibu, the place where tourists, surfers, diners, and fishermen all vie for the same parking places,

Malibu Pier and Escondido Beach

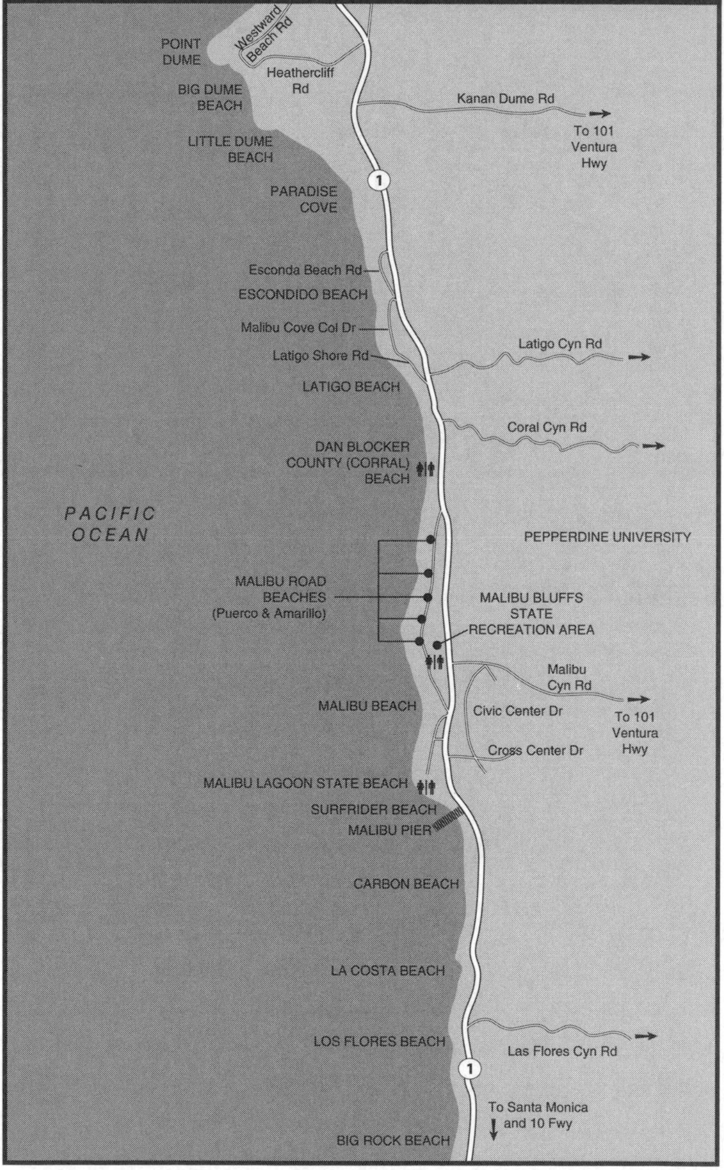

is at **Malibu Pier.** For paddlers who enjoy people-watching more than they enjoy solitude, there are a couple of SUP rental operations on Pacific Coast Highway and a small launch space just south of the pilings. Probably the easiest parking here is in the $10 city lot, but there is also free parallel parking on Pacific Coast Highway—you'll just have to fight the surfers for a space. Paddling near the pier allows for distant L.A. city views and close-up views of some of the area's prized beachfront real estate. North of the pier is **Malibu Point,** the famed surf break that spawned the reputations of Gidget and Mickey Dora (to name a few). The break is always famously crowded and probably not the best spot for stand-up paddlers, particularly those without surfing experience. Probably the best nearby option for paddlers is to head south of the pier toward the waterfront homes at **Carbon Beach.** But for those who want to do a more substantial paddle in less congested waters, I suggest heading farther north.

Escondido Beach lies roughly 5.5 miles north of the Malibu Pier and just south of Geoffrey's Malibu restaurant. Parking is a bit tricky, but there is space for about 20 cars to park parallel on the southbound side of Pacific Coast Highway. The beach access is via a gate between Malibu Cove Colony Drive and Escondido Beach Road. (There is another beach access north of Geoffrey's Malibu, but paddlers will find it nearly impossible to haul their boards down the narrow staircase.)

On a sunny weekday in late summer, the small beach in front of Escondido Creek was mostly uncrowded. The sunbathers who do come here know enough to avoid the $40 parking fee at nearby **Paradise Cove.** Even though the surf was particularly large, the launch and landing at Escondido Beach weren't too difficult. The waves break close to the shore, so it's fairly easy to push out beyond the surf zone. My plan was to paddle north to Paradise Cove. The beach with the expensive parking has a popular restaurant and a pier. It's also one of the more scenic spots on the Malibu coast—a nice sandy beach just leeward of the cliffs of **Point Dume.**

Unfortunately, my paddle was cut short a bit by a stiff headwind. I had left too late in the afternoon, and the westerlies were blowing fairly strong. In calmer conditions, one could easily paddle to Paradise Cove in 30–40 minutes. You can't launch there, however, because the owners of the Paradise Cove Beach Cafe control all access to the beach and refuse to allow boards to come through (although the California Coastal Commission is currently challenging this policy, as well as the exorbitant parking fee).

Save the wind, you have few obstacles to approaching Paradise Cove from the water: Just paddle up to the beach near the pier and, if you like, enjoy a nice lunch at the restaurant. Continuing north of Paradise, it's about a mile to the reef-lined cove of **Little Dume.** Just past this cove one finds the rugged beaches and cliffs of Point Dume. Obviously, I haven't paddled these waters, but based on photos and reputation, this is an area that is definitely worth exploring—and one I hope to return to.

DIRECTIONS AND PARKING The Malibu Pier is 9 miles north of Santa Monica on Pacific Coast Highway. Free parking is available on PCH, but it can be difficult to procure a spot. Those launching SUP boards would probably do well to park in the lot next to the pier ($10 flat rate).

Escondido Beach is another 5.5 miles north of the pier. Park on the southbound shoulder of Pacific Coast Highway, just south of Geoffrey's Malibu, and walk down the highway to the access gate, between Malibu Cove Colony Drive and Escondido Beach Road.

Parking at Paradise Cove costs a whopping $40, or $6 with a voucher from the Paradise Cove Beach Cafe. The owners of the property are fighting with the California Coastal Commission to maintain a ban on launching boards at the beach. In 2015, however, the **Stand Up for Clean Water Paddleboard Race** was held at Paradise Cove.

RENTALS AND LESSONS Tony Stearns at **Radfish Malibu** (310-433-1767, **radfishmalibu.com**) has a mobile operation and provides rentals and lessons at several Malibu locations, including the pier and

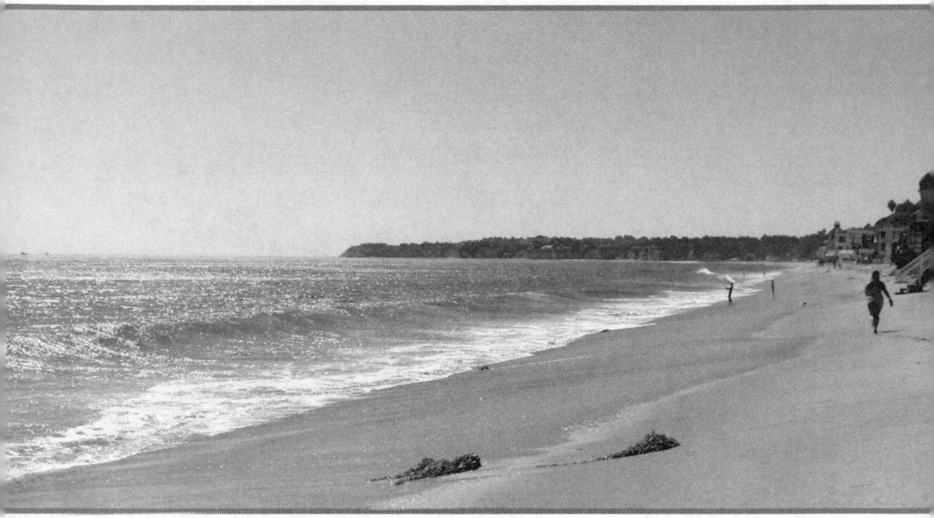

Looking down Escondido Beach

Escondido Beach. He also sells and shapes boards (including some that are built by hand in Malibu). Tony offers a free SUP lesson with every board purchase.

Malibu Surf Shack (22935 Pacific Coast Highway; 310-456-8508, **malibusurfshack.com**) is a rental house and surf shop just across PCH from the Malibu Pier. SUP rentals run $45 for 2 hours and $55 for 4 hours.

BEACH-ACCESS INFORMATION The **Los Angeles Urban Rangers** is a group committed to exploring and maintaining public easements along the Malibu coastline. Their two-page PDF beach guide (**tinyurl.com/malibubeachguide**) details every legal entry point along the 27-mile stretch.

Leo Carrillo State Park

Malibu

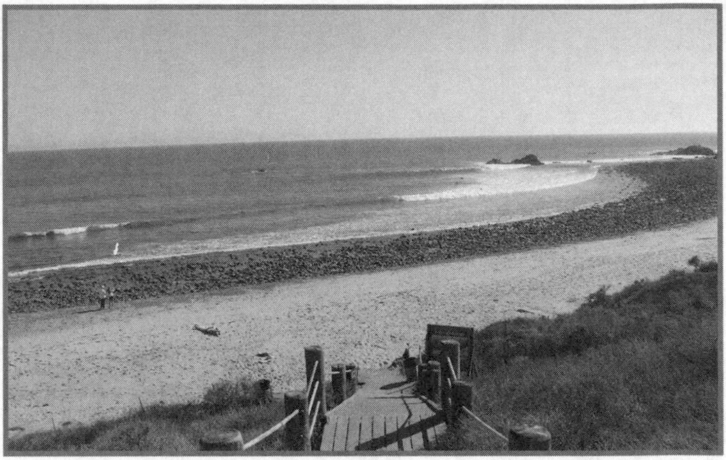

The rock-strewn shoreline at South Beach in Leo Carrillo State Park

OVERVIEW Leo Carrillo State Park lies about 20 minutes north of the Malibu Pier, in the heart of the Santa Monica Mountains National Recreation Area. It's one of the most picture-perfect beaches in Southern California. If you don't believe me, just ask any Hollywood location scout. The state beach has been a popular filming location for more than 60 years, providing a backdrop to movies like *Gidget, The Karate Kid, Point Break, Grease,* and many others.

Productions come to Leo because it's the prototypical idyllic California beach. Above the sand and the blue Pacific are wide-open and undeveloped hillsides. It's a scene reminiscent of old California: the coastal paradise that existed before sprawl and smog and gridlock.

The state beach may be off the beaten path, but that doesn't mean it isn't popular. Leo attracts a fairly regular crowd of surfers, windsurfers, and beachgoers. Camping spaces in the nearby canyon are some of the most sought-after in the state park system. If you want to reserve a summer weekend spot, you need to do so several months in advance.

WHERE TO PADDLE **Sequit Point** divides the coastal portion of the park, and the two beaches on either side are aptly named **North Beach**

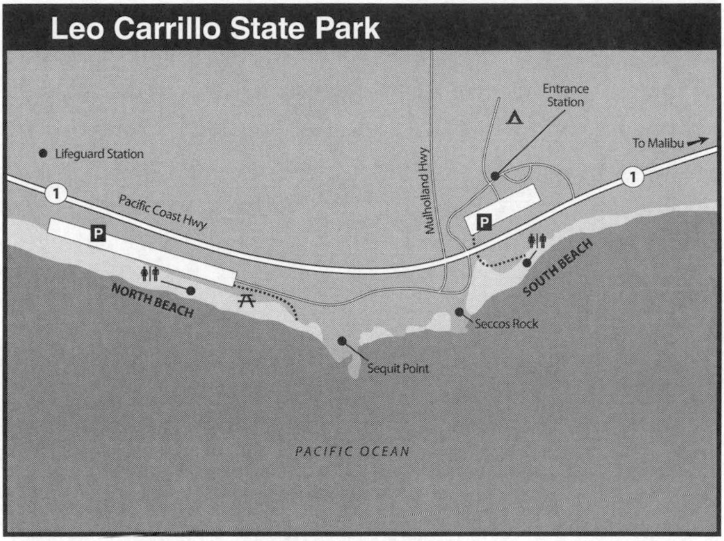

and **South Beach.** Most paddlers will want to launch at North Beach, simply because there are far fewer rocks along the shoreline and the beach offers better parking options. The only downside is that North Beach has more exposure to west winds (the inside waters at South Beach are protected by the point).

The parking lot at North Beach abuts the long, sandy strand above Sequit Point. The beach is exposed to surf, but the waves typically break close to shore. On the day I paddled here, it was pretty easy to get through the medium-sized surf, but there was a bit of chop from the wind. I headed north, windward, trying to find smooth water to the lee of the kelp paddies. From the water, there were panoramic views of the tawny-hued shore cliffs, the steep rise of the Santa Monica Mountains, and distant Point Mugu. The scenery almost made up for the difficult headwind.

Continuing northwest, past North Beach, there is another sandy strand, which terminates at a rock-strewn point. Here, atop a sea wall, is the **Malibu Bay Club,** an exclusive beachfront community that sits between the state beach and **County Line Beach.** Outside this point are several kelp-lined reefs, which, under most conditions, merely provide a bit of bump in the ocean swells, and not breaking waves. Closer inside, more-consistent waves roll around the rocky point. (This should be of particular note to stand-up surfers.) The stretch between the Malibu Bay Club and North Beach has a few off-the-beaten-path surf breaks. On a less bumpy day (less windy than when I was there), these peaks might be fun to check out. Not too many prone surfers come here because of the lack of convenient access. This is in contrast with County Line, the sandy beach just on the other side of the exclusive community, which tends to attract a substantial crew of surfers.

Because of the wind, I decided not to continue toward County Line, and instead turned around and made the easy paddle back to the car. I wish I could have paddled more, because when conditions permit, there is plenty to explore along the stretch. The offshore reefs and kelp paddies are excellent for diving and fishing, and for stand-up surfers, the relatively isolated beaches have the potential to produce fun, uncrowded waves. For those who simply want to paddle, the coast near Leo Carrillo offers amazing views and beautiful open water. The trick is simply to avoid that pesky wind.

During spring and summer, the wind blows fairly consistently at Leo Carrillo. The steep rise of the Santa Monica Mountains creates a venturi effect, accelerating the afternoon sea breezes as they head down the coast from Point Mugu toward Point Dume. Typically, the westerlies build throughout the afternoon, culminating late in the day with so-called sundowner winds. So if you want to paddle this stretch of coast, it's best to paddle early in the day. The other option is to do a downwind paddle ending at Leo Carrillo. This requires two cars and a certain level of confidence and experience, but it can be a fun way to see the coast. Depending on how far you want to paddle, there are several places to set out. County Line would be the closest place to start, but if you want a longer downwind paddle, you could launch from **Sycamore Canyon** or from **Point Mugu State Park.** The latter beach is 7 miles north of Leo Carrillo and also serves as the starting point for the **Malibu Downwinder.** Held each year in May, the race begins at Point Mugu and finishes at North Beach. The event is open to stand-up paddlers and prone paddlers of varying ages and abilities. There's also a nice beach barbecue at the finish (I've included information on the next page).

South Beach at Leo Carrillo is also quite beautiful, but the shoreline is littered with bread loaf–sized rocks. On the upside, free parking is available nearby on the southbound side of Pacific Coast Highway. (On the other hand, it may be worth paying the park entrance fee in order to avoid the agony of the feet.) If you're determined to paddle here, try launching at high tide. Park parallel on Pacific Coast Highway just south of the park entrance, and access the beach via the staircase. There may be fewer rocks south of the staircase, but don't count on it.

The point at South Beach is a popular surfing break, with a long right-peeling wave that forms off **Secos Rock.** Unfortunately, stand-up surfing is not allowed here. There are signs on the beach detailing the surfing boundaries. Stand-up surfers should launch in the windsurfing and kayaking areas (which begin roughly in front of the staircase). There is a significant offshore reef just south of the point (either submerged or above the water level depending on the tide), and farther outside are some fairly dense kelp paddies. If you paddle beyond the point, be prepared to encounter some strong, gusty winds. Also, when paddling back to shore, be aware of the rocks in shallow water. There are plenty of opportunities to nick—or even break—your leg, which is not a fun way to end your paddle.

DIRECTIONS AND PARKING Leo Carrillo State Park is on Pacific Coast Highway, 28 miles north of Santa Monica. Driving north on PCH, continue about a mile past Nicholas Canyon, and turn right off the highway to enter the park. To get to North Beach, follow the park road past the South Beach parking lot and continue under the highway, following the road until you reach your destination. Parking is $10 for day use. Annual passes for California State Parks cost $195.

You can find free parking along the southbound shoulder of Pacific Coast Highway, but for those wanting to paddle from North Beach, entering the state park is advisable (it's a pretty long walk from the highway to the beach). For those who want to paddle at South Beach, the closest parking is along the highway.

FACILITIES There are restrooms and outdoor showers at North Beach. The state park also has a popular campground; call 800-444-7275 or check **reserveamerica.com** for reservations and availability.

CONDITIONS AND HAZARDS If the surf is large, expect some moderate shore pound at North Beach. There are some rocks along the shoreline, but not nearly as many as at South Beach. Wind is often an issue here. In the summer months, when the San Fernando Valley heats up and the coast is cool, thermal winds will kick up in the afternoon.

NATURAL FEATURES Look for some nice walk-in caves and tidepools in and around Sequit Point. The caves and rock features, which have been used as backdrops for several films and TV shows, make for some fun post-paddle beachcombing.

MALIBU DOWNWINDER This race begins at Point Mugu and ends at North Beach, where a barbecue and awards ceremony are held. The event has been going on since 2004 and is typically held on the first weekend in May. Visit **malibudw.blogspot.com** for more information.

Ventura and Santa Barbara Counties

Tranquil conditions at Refugio State Beach (see page 144)

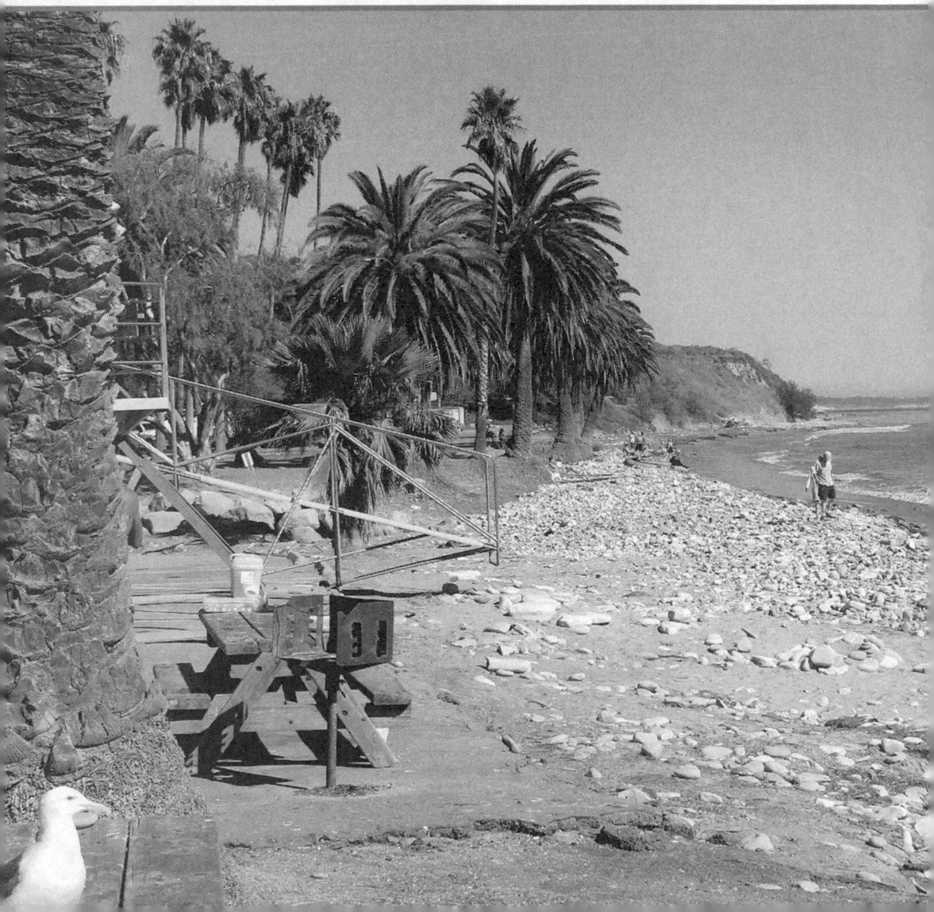

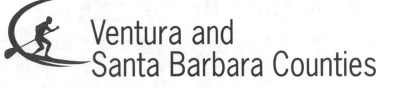

Harbor Cove Beach **Ventura**

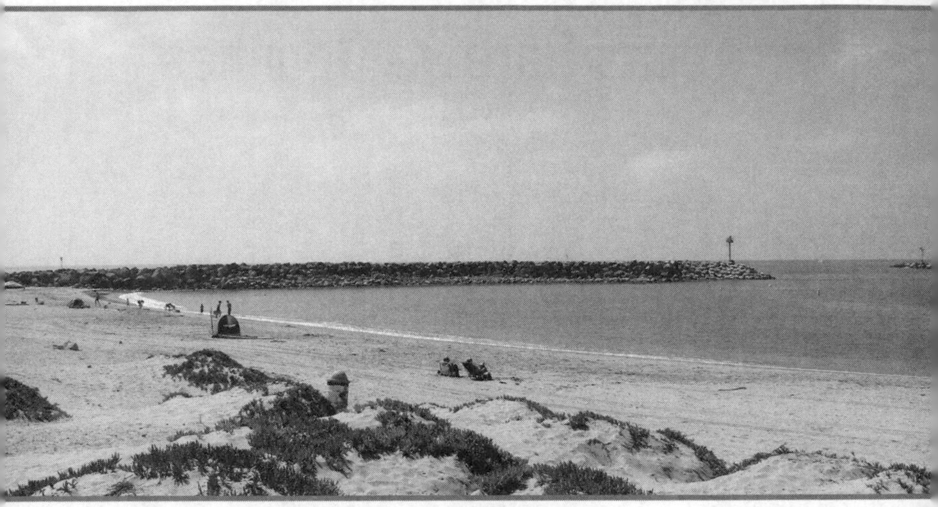

The calm and inviting waters at Harbor Cove Beach

OVERVIEW The sandy beach at Harbor Cove lies near the edge of Ventura Harbor, just inside of the marina's three prominent rock jetties. The jetties effectively block swells from every direction, forming a cocoon of protective water. Although there is significant surf on the other side of the South Jetty, nary a wave reaches Harbor Cove. For anyone who wants to cruise around in flat, calm water, this is the place to go. And for those who want the opportunity to paddle in a variety of conditions, it's only about a 10-minute paddle past the South Jetty.

WHERE TO PADDLE Parking at the cove is free and fairly abundant. There are spaces within a few feet of the sand. A short trek from the car takes one to the calm water at the shoreline. Ventura posts lifeguards here in the summer, but I can't imagine they make many rescues. This beach is perfect for families—parents should feel safe letting their children paddle at Harbor Cove. Moreover, just about anyone who wants a drama-free SUP experience will appreciate the cove's easy access and launch.

Once you're out on the water, you'll have plenty of space to explore. If you don't wish to paddle in the open ocean, you have the

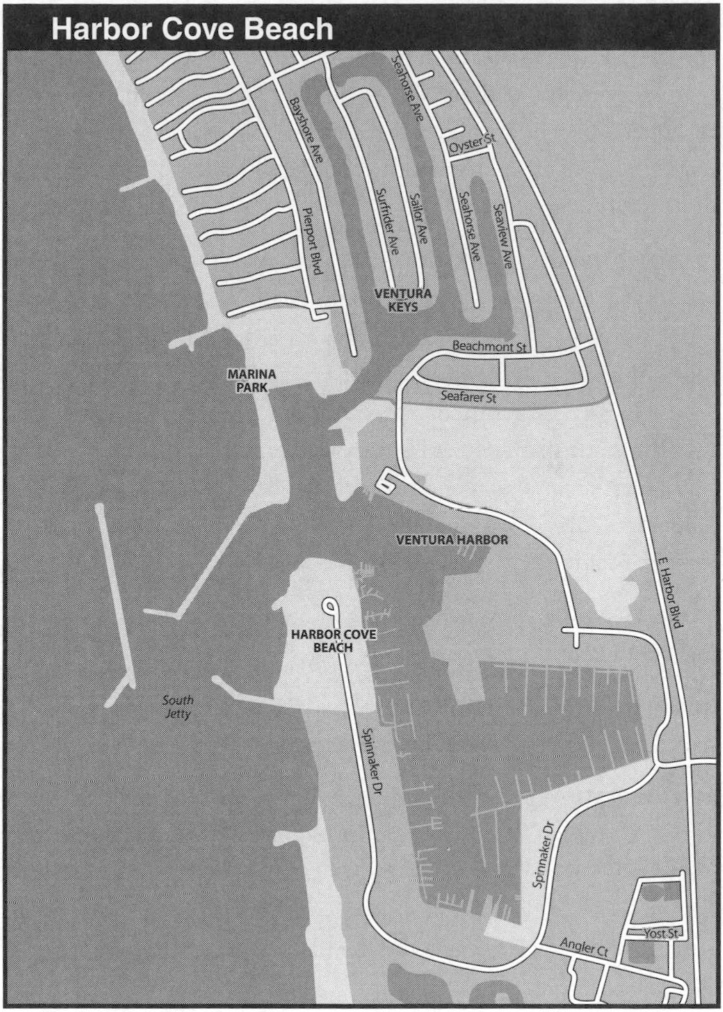

entire harbor to the east and the **Ventura Keys** to the north (the keys are narrow boating channels lined with homes and docks). To get to the keys, head north and then northeast across the channel, passing the entrance to Ventura Harbor. Continue north and inside of **Marina Park;** eventually, you'll see the entrance to the keys over your right shoulder (to the northeast). From here, it's possible to do a lap around the two parallel channels before returning to Harbor Cove.

Those without their own equipment should check out **Paddlesurf Outlet.** They offer appointment-based lessons and rentals at Harbor Cove. Just meet them in the parking lot and go (see below for more information).

DIRECTIONS AND PARKING From I-101 southbound, take the Seaward Avenue exit, then turn left onto East Harbor Boulevard. After roughly 2 miles, turn right on Spinnaker Drive. Continue another 2 miles around the harbor until you reach the Harbor Cove parking lot.

From I-101 northbound, exit at South Victoria Avenue, then turn left (south). After 0.6 mile, turn right onto Olivas Park Drive, then continue straight. Upon entering the harbor, Olivas Park will become Spinnaker Drive. Drive around the harbor for another 2 miles until you reach the Harbor Cove parking lot. Parking is free.

FACILITIES There are restrooms and outdoor showers in the parking lot at Harbor Cove.

CONDITIONS AND HAZARDS The cove is well protected and family-friendly. Dogs are welcome on the beach.

RENTALS AND LESSONS Although their shop is located a few miles east in Camarillo, **Paddlesurf Outlet** (805-415-7674, **paddlesurfoutlet.com**) offers lessons, rentals, and board demonstrations at Harbor Cove (as well as Channel Islands Harbor). Rentals run $39 for 2 hours. Just call for an appointment and they'll meet you in the parking lot.

SANTA BARBARA BEACHES

Santa Barbara

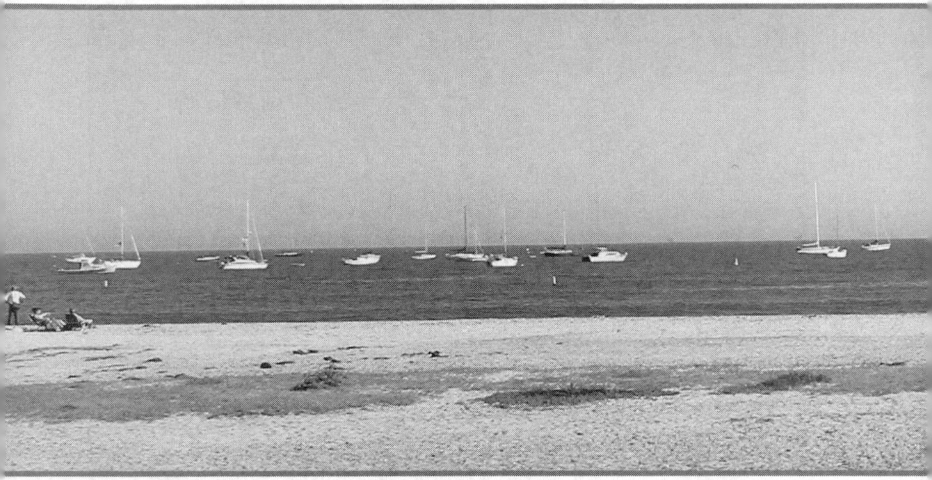

Boats moored in the lee of Stearns Wharf at East Beach

OVERVIEW This mild-mannered resort town has an active and dedicated community of stand-up paddlers. And it's easy to see why. Sheltered by the steep rise of the Santa Ynez Mountains, Santa Barbara enjoys fairly mild weather year-round. Although the outer waters along the Santa Barbara channel tend to be windy, the near-shore waters, inside the barrier of the Channel Islands, tend to be calm. There are plenty of glassy days along the Santa Barbara coast, and the city has several beaches that offer paddlers a variety of conditions, from flat-water to peeling waves. Consequently, Santa Barbara can be an ideal place to learn stand-up paddling, as well as a fun destination for seasoned SUPers.

WHERE TO PADDLE Close to downtown, **East Beach** and **West Beach** lie on either side of the large pier known as **Stearns Wharf.** (The city of Santa Barbara faces south, so the coastline runs east to west.) The long sand strand at East Beach tends be the most popular beach in Santa Barbara. From the parking lot, it's a bit of a walk to the water, but launching is easy in the shadow of the pier. Stearns Wharf, once a terminal for passengers and freight, is now a tourist attraction lined

with restaurants and shops. From the water, you can watch the activity on the pier. You might even be able to catch glimpses of tourists feeding some of the world's largest pelicans (or if not the largest, then definitely the most gluttonous). In the lee of the wharf are a collection of moored boats and a calm stretch of water that, aside from an occasional bit of boat wake, makes for perfect stress-free paddling. This is a great place to cruise around, enjoy the sun, and take in the scenery.

On the other side of the pier, **Santa Barbara Harbor** provides the simplest access to West Beach. Look for the boat ramp near the **Santa Barbara Sailing Center.** This is an easy, almost fail-safe launch for beginners. The harbor is also a staging area for SUP yoga classes, as well as general SUP lessons. A short paddle from the launch takes you outside the harbor and into the calm waters between West Beach and Stearns Wharf.

A surf break known as **Sandspit** lies just west of the harbor mouth. Experienced paddlers may think about paddling out to this break on small surf days—when the surf gets big, Sandspit becomes

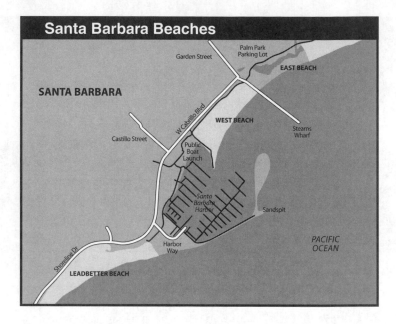

fast, hollow, and prone to a dramatic backwash effect. On these days, the break definitely won't be appropriate for stand-up boards, but it might be fun to watch from a distance.

Farther west is **Leadbetter Beach,** a small, cliff-lined strand that's popular with stand-up surfers. As with most Santa Barbara surf spots, this right-breaking point will definitely be better in winter, but Leadbetter produces some waves even on smaller summer days. It's not a fast wave, but it wraps nicely around the point allowing for long rides. Leadbetter can get crowded because it's close to town. Otherwise, it's a nice beach with convenient parking, restrooms, and outdoor showers.

For those who want to escape the tourist-centric beaches near downtown, **Butterfly Beach** in nearby Montecito is a nice alternative. Just east of the Four Seasons Resort, this section of coast is popular with local beachgoers and dog owners (dogs are welcome off-leash). Butterfly Beach has limited parking (on the adjacent street), so paddlers should try to arrive early. The beach also lacks any facilities or restrooms, but it is scenic and nice for paddling. Look for smooth surface conditions inside the barrier of offshore kelp paddies; if you're lucky, you might run across a pod of passing dolphins.

Just east of the resort is a fickle point break known as **Hammond's.** On rare days when it has large surf, Hammond's will be crowded with an aggressive crew of local surfers. On smaller days, it will be less crowded (if it's even breaking, that is), but you may want to talk to other local stand-up paddlers before surfing this break on your board.

For other paddling locations near Santa Barbara, see the next two sections, on Goleta Beach and Refugio State Beach, respectively. Whether you live here or just plan to visit, there is plenty of accessible coastline just waiting to be explored. With amazing scenery and calm water, Santa Barbara is a world-class location for stand-up paddling.

DIRECTIONS AND PARKING East Beach is just off East Cabrillo Boulevard (in the 200 block, near Garden Street). Parking is available in the Palm Park parking lot at $2 per hour. Limited free street parking is also available at the south end of Santa Barbara Street (near the train tracks, about a two-block walk from the sand).

The parking lot for West Beach and Santa Barbara Harbor is in the 300 block of West Cabrillo Boulevard. The public launch in the harbor is just west of the Santa Barbara Sailing Center. Parking runs $2 per hour and $12 per day.

Leadbetter Beach lies 0.3 mile west of West Beach at 800 Shoreline Drive (West Cabrillo Boulevard becomes Shoreline Drive as you pass the harbor). Parking is available in the Shoreline lot for $2 per hour. Just east of the beach are additional spots in the West Harbor lot. Here, parking runs $3 for 3 hours and $7 per day.

Butterfly Beach is in Montecito, roughly 5 miles east of downtown Santa Barbara. To get there, take US 101 south and exit at Olive Mill Road. After exiting, take the first right on Olive Mill Road and then another immediate right on Hill Road. Follow Hill for 0.5 mile and make a right onto Butterfly Lane. There is limited free street parking (perhaps 50 spaces) on Butterfly Lane.

RENTALS, LESSONS, AND YOGA Two blocks from East Beach, **Stand Up Paddle Sports** (121 Santa Barbara St.; 888-805-9978 or 805-962-7877; **supsports.com**) was the first dedicated SUP shop in North

Stearns Wharf

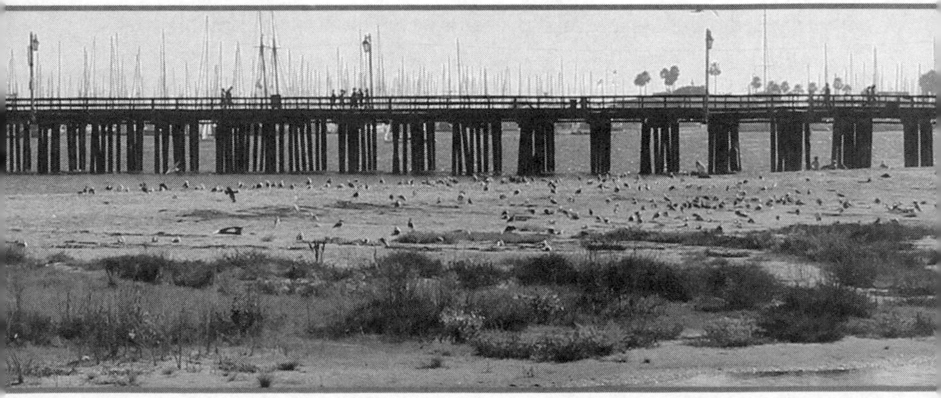

America, and they're still going strong. They have a knowledgeable staff and a full line of boards shaped and manufactured under their own label. Rentals from the shop run $20 for 1 hour, $35 for 2 hours, $50 for a half-day, and $75 for a full day. Lessons cost $75, and are generally held at West Beach.

The **Santa Barbara Sailing Center** (805-962-2826, **sbsail.com**) has beginner boards, foam boards, and a few performance boards for rent at its location in Santa Barbara Harbor, next to the boat ramp. Basic boards rent for $15 per hour, performance boards $30 per hour. They also offer 2-hour guided tours for $50 per person (two-person minimum).

Channel Islands Outfitters (117-B Harbor Way; 805-617-3425, **paddlesportsca.com**) has a paddling center in the harbor where they offer board rentals and lessons.

From June to September, **Santa Barbara Fitness Tours** (805-628-2444, **santabarbarafitnesstours.com**) offers SUP yoga classes at West Beach in front of the Hotel Milo (202 W. Cabrillo Blvd.).

LOCAL BURRITO OK, truth be told, there are no burritos to be had at **La Super-Rica** (622 N. Milpas St.; 805-963-4940), but this taqueria serves some of the best Mexican food on the planet. Hyperbole, you say? Just ask the crowd lined up on Milpas Street waiting to get in. Or ask *Sunset* magazine, which named it "the world's best taco joint." Unfortunately, you can't ask Julia Child anymore, but late in life the French gastronomy expert championed La Super-Rica.

Locals may tell you it's overrated. They may recommend some other hole-in-the-wall that might be less crowded and less expensive. Well, they're wrong. As you walk in the front door, you can see the cooks making fresh tortillas and roasted peppers to order. And you can see the expectation on the customers' faces. Try one of the daily specials or any of the tacos. Have some fresh guacamole and maybe a *horchata*. Splurge. You waited a long time, and it's all good.

Goleta Beach County Park

Goleta

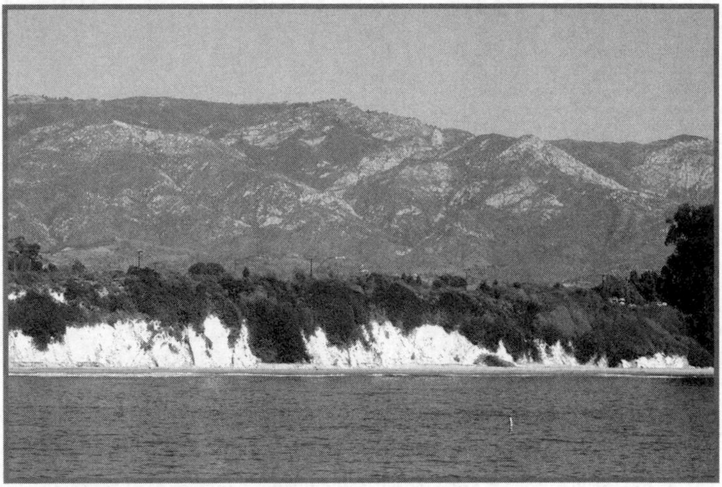

The distant Santa Ynez Mountains viewed from Goleta Beach

OVERVIEW Every time I see the campus at UC Santa Barbara, I wonder why I didn't go to college there. Built on the bluffs of scenic Goleta Point, the university looks more like a tony resort than a college campus. Students attend classes in buildings that are, perhaps, a Frisbee throw from the high-tide line. The school has its own beach and its own estuary. There's even a surf break named Campus Point.

Unfortunately, for myself and many others, it's too late to attend UCSB, but we can always paddle the tranquil waters near the campus. Goleta Beach County Park, which lies just south of the campus, is one of the more popular beaches for Santa Barbara stand-up paddlers. And it's easy to see why. The beach park offers free parking close to the water and a smooth, sandy beach for launching SUP boards. Other amenities include a pier, a restaurant, and a nice shaded lawn with picnic tables and restrooms. The surf at Goleta tends to be small and gentle.

WHERE TO PADDLE I recommend launching north of the pier and paddling up toward the campus. North of the beach park, pale cliffs border the grounds of the university, extending all the way to

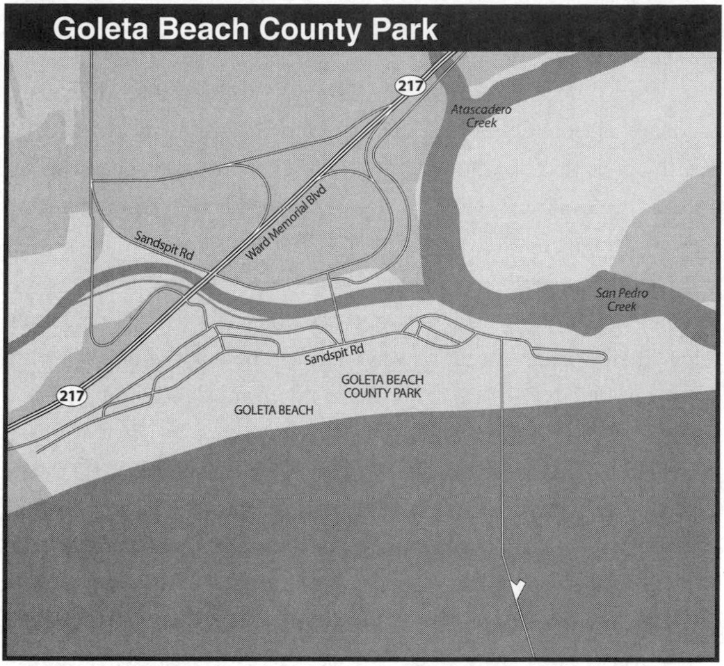

Goleta Point (also known as **Campus Point**). These waters also form the boundary of the **Campus Point State Marine Conservation Area,** a protected area of coastline that extends up the coast to **Coal Oil Point Reserve.** (I suppose "Coal Oil Point Marine Conservation Area" would have sounded too ridiculously paradoxical.) The conservation area is designed to maintain the habitat for the diverse collection of marine life that frequents these waters. California sea otters can be found here—it's their southernmost habitat—as well as migrating gray whales, sea lions, dolphins, and shorebirds. On the day I paddled here, I saw a few sea lions and plenty of diving pelicans.

It takes about 30 minutes to paddle up to Campus Point. Inside the point is a small, protected cove that is understandably popular with the local student population. There is also surf here, and depending on the tide, the break can be fun stand-up surfing. When I was here, there was one SUP surfer in the cove, but the conditions were small and bumpy.

Past Campus Point is **Isla Vista,** a cliff-lined strand that extends up to Coal Oil Point. The reefs outside the latter, lined with healthy beds of kelp and eelgrass, offer excellent opportunities for snorkeling (obviously, fishing is not allowed due to the protected status of the waters).

During a south-wind day, I found the water conditions outside of Campus Point a bit rough from chop, which made for difficult paddling. There was also a bit of wave refraction near the point, which, when combined with the chop, made my board dance around like a cork. However, local SUPers will tell you that there are plenty of calm days here. When the weather cooperates, the paddle to Isla Vista can be quite nice and quite rewarding. It's a beautiful stretch of water—scenic and teeming with avian and marine life. From the water, there are also unobstructed views of the dramatic peaks of the Santa Ynez Mountains. And on clear days, it's possible to see distant **Santa Cruz Island.**

Even if you stay at one of the picturesque beaches near downtown Santa Barbara, I recommend making the drive up to Goleta Beach. For those without boards, there is an on-site SUP rental facility inside the county park, so getting out on the water is a snap. Then, once you start paddling, the beautiful views from UCSB will be right in front of you. Just remember—renting, or even buying, an SUP board is much less expensive than making college-tuition payments.

DIRECTIONS AND PARKING From downtown Santa Barbara, take US 101 north, then take CA 217 west toward UCSB. After 1.8 miles, exit at Sandspit Road. Turn left and then stay on Sandspit Road (don't go to the university) until you reach the entrance for Goleta Beach County Park. Parking is free. I recommend the spaces close to Beachside Bar-Cafe (at the pier).

CONDITIONS AND HAZARDS Summer tends to bring calm conditions here, so paddling at Goleta is generally safe and easy. The beach and shore are sandy, and the waves tend to be small. On south-wind days, it may be difficult to paddle outside of Campus Point. Also, in the spring and summer, this beach (and particularly Isla Vista) may be prone to late afternoon sundowner winds.

FACILITIES Fairly clean restrooms and outdoor showers, plus a shaded grass area with picnic tables.

ATTRACTIONS The wildlife here includes marine mammals, diving birds, and college students.

RENTALS **Channel Islands Outfitters** (805-617-3425, **paddlesportsca.com**) runs a paddle-sports center at Goleta Beach (5986 Sandspit Road; you'll pass it as you drive in). They offer a decent selection of boards, and they take reservations by phone. SUP rentals run $40 for 2 hours and $100 for 24 hours.

If you're driving from downtown, you may want to talk to the folks at **Stand Up Paddle Sports** (121 Santa Barbara St.; 888-805-9978 or 805-962-7877; **supsports.com**). This is the largest shop in Santa Barbara and one of the most established shops in Southern California.

LOCAL BURRITO Started by a couple of hippies, **Freebirds World Burrito** (879 Embarcadero Road; 805-968-0123, **freebirds.com**) offers large portions and (fairly) healthy ingredients. It's a UCSB institution, so be prepared: If you're over 25, you could be the oldest person in the Isla Vista restaurant. If you come here late on a Friday night, don't expect anyone to be sober. The burritos are good, if not great, and they have a nice selection of salsas, including roasted corn with jalapeño.

Refugio State Beach **Goleta**

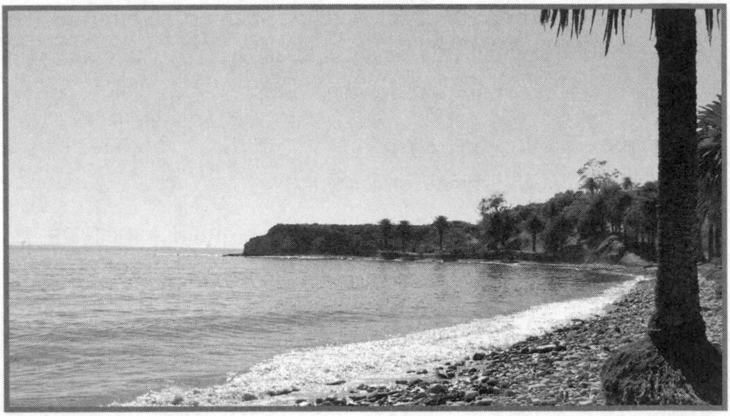

The tree-lined cove at Refugio State Beach

OVERVIEW Heading north from Santa Barbara, Highway 101 hugs the coast for several miles before veering inland behind the dramatic rise of Point Conception. Along this scenic stretch are three state beach parks: El Capitán, Refugio, and Gaviota. Of the three, Refugio and El Capitán are good for stand-up paddling, while Gaviota tends to be prone to fierce offshore winds. (A localized effect: Northwest winds whip inside Point Conception and then funnel down the canyon toward Gaviota.).

WHERE TO PADDLE The protected cove at Refugio State Beach is tranquil and quaint, with palm trees near the shore and picnic tables shaded by the fronds. The beach is quite narrow, and the shoreline trees grow only a few feet beyond the high-tide line. On the day I paddled here, the surf was, per usual, quite small, and the beach looked more like a lakeshore than the edge of the Pacific. It's possible to park within 50 feet of the tideline—remarkable for an ocean beach—so getting out into the water is fast and effortless. Cobblestones are mixed with the sand along the shore, but because of the typically calm conditions, launching tends to be easy.

I made the short paddle out of the cove, following the cliff-lined shore and heading north in the direction of **Point Conception.** Beyond

the cove, there is no real water access, as the ocean washes into sharp cliffs. The secluded coast here has a network of shallow reefs that sustain a robust collection of sea life. As I peered down through the kelp and submerged rocks, I spied several schools of small fish—probably anchovies—and once I was met by a passing pod of dolphins, which were attracted to the bait balls.

Heading north, the scenery doesn't vary much, but it doesn't have to. Near the cliffs, one gets a feeling of seclusion, a feeling that is interrupted only by squawking seagulls and the rush of the tide against the rocks. Because it's in the shadow of Point Conception, the water tends to be calm here, but because there isn't a beach, waves do push back off the cliff, creating a bit of backwash that might challenge some paddlers. This effect should be less prevalent at lower tides; if it's a problem, one can always paddle a bit farther offshore to find more stable surface conditions.

Returning to the cove, you'll encounter a small point break that sometimes produces waves. (It's pretty fickle. El Capitán is generally a better bet for those who want to stand-up surf.) And inside of the point, a bit of rocky shoreline is popular with fishermen. The smooth

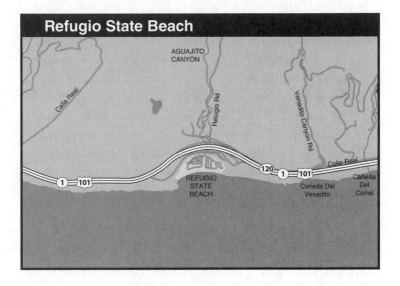

water inside the cove is perfect for beginner SUPers, and just about every paddler will appreciate the calm conditions at the shoreline.

As you return to the beach, it's tempting to relax under the shade of the trees. Although the highway may be just up the canyon, it feels miles away. There is a small general store in the parking lot, but the facilities at the state beach are a bit rustic. That just adds to the appeal, though. Refugio feels like a beach stuck in another era. It's a perfect place to get out and cruise around on an SUP board, then sit on the sand and enjoy a peaceful afternoon.

DIRECTIONS AND PARKING From downtown Santa Barbara, follow US 101 for 22 miles and exit at Refugio Road. Turn left and follow the road to the state park. Past the entrance, head to the day-use area at the north end of the cove. There is beachfront parking near the general store and the basketball courts. Day-use parking is $10; annual passes for California State Parks cost $195.

FACILITIES There are restrooms nearby and a nice area for picnicking or just lying around, but not, as far as I could tell, any outdoor showers (the campground has enclosed coin-operated showers). A small store near the launch sells snacks and camping provisions.

CONDITIONS AND HAZARDS The surf tends to be calm here, and west winds are often blocked by Point Conception. There are some stones on the shore, but it's fairly easy to get past them. Outside the cove, the ocean pushes up against cliffs, creating some wave refraction. Also, paddling outside the cove means heading into fairly remote waters, so, as always, be safe and be frank about your abilities and limitations.

EL CAPITÁN STATE BEACH Three miles south of Refugio, El Capitán has day-use and camping spots. Park on the bluff north of the point and access the water via a short staircase. The beach is nice for paddling, and down at the point there tends to be a small, soft wave that can be fun for stand-up paddling. On the rare days when large west swells wrap around Point Conception, the point at El Capitán transforms into a magical (and perhaps crowded) surf spot.

Stand-Up Surfing

SURFING MAY BE one of the most exciting and dynamic activities to do on an SUP board, but before you take your board into the lineup, you need to understand the rules of the game. What follows is a brief discussion about surfing conditions and culture, as well as some tips on how to maximize your surfing experience.

Your Board Is Big: A Simple Primer on Surf Etiquette

PERHAPS YOU'VE SEEN glossy videos of stand-up surfing. There are plenty of them out there: smartly edited pieces featuring stand-up surfers carving turns and sharing waves with groups of prone surfers. In surfer parlance, everyone is stoked—smiling for the camera and happy to be out on the water.

In real life, however, the scenario may be a bit different. If you paddle your SUP board out to a crowded surf break, your reception may be less than friendly. Depending on the beach, the reaction of the surfers may range from disdainful disregard to outright anger and even aggressive behavior. Many surfers have a proprietary relationship with their favorite break—they don't want more surfers there, they don't want new surfers there, and they certainly don't want someone with a paddle surfing there.

You may dismiss this possessive stance as self-centered and immature, but there are realities that give rise to it. Crowds are definitely a factor in busy Southern California. There is a finite number of surfable waves, and plenty of people who want to surf them. Surfing is rarely an egalitarian experience; talented and experienced surfers often get the lion's share of the waves. Nevertheless, all surfers are expected to abide by the rules of surfing etiquette (the most important rule being not to drop in on someone who's already on a wave). Newcomers not only add to the crowds but may also be perceived as ignorant of the rules of surfing or the nuances of the break. And if you're a newcomer on an SUP board, you have the added stigma of being on a large, cumbersome, and possibly dangerous board.

Not to defend anyone's poor attitude, but SUP boards create a few particular concerns for surfers:

1. Aided by a paddle, these large boards are capable of catching waves earlier than traditional boards. This changes the dynamic of the lineup. Depending on the break, a group of stand-up surfers can completely dominate a lineup of prone surfers, hogging every wave.
2. Because they have more weight and volume, SUP boards can be dangerous in the surf. Of course, this is relative—some stand-up surfboards are smaller and lighter than longboards—but the danger still exists.
3. Inexperienced stand-up surfers may not know how to control their boards in the surf. This is really an extension of the previous concern, but it deserves special consideration. Maneuvering an SUP board down a wave and through a pack of surfers requires a certain level of competence. Being unable to turn the board or falling off the board at inopportune times may result in collisions, damaged equipment, and even injuries. Even when you're paddling out on your board, there can be dangers. If you get caught inside of breaking waves, you may find it difficult to hold onto your board. And if the board drags behind you—even if it's on a leash—it can hit other surfers in the water.

As a beginning stand-up surfer, you must respect other surfers and keep yourself and others safe. It's best to make your first attempts at stand-up surfing on an open section of beach, away from other surfers and paddlers. While you're learning, you don't need the best break, just a wave to practice on.

Before you paddle out into a crowded lineup, it's important that you acquire some basic competence in the waves. To a certain degree, you should know how to turn your board on the wave face, how to drop in on a wave without pearling, how to pull back out of waves you've already started paddling for, and how to control your board when caught inside of the breaking waves. None of these skills are learned overnight, so as you progress in the sport, it may be best to seek out breaks with designated SUP boundaries—or at least breaks that have unofficial SUP zones. Learning around other stand-up surfers will definitely be more encouraging.

Surfers tend to be passionate about their pastime, and they have to be: It takes commitment to learn how to ride waves and even more time on the water to master the sport. Be respectful of that commitment by following these guidelines.

Use common sense. When paddling out, stay clear of the section of the wave where people are surfing—paddle around the break until you're safely outside the impact zone. If you see a pack of surfers sharing one peak, try to find another wave of your own. Remember that one of the advantages of being on a stand-up board is that you can catch waves that are inaccessible to many prone surfers.

Know your ability. If you sense you aren't going to be able to maneuver your board through the lineup and maintain control of your board when caught inside, then trust your instincts and consider a different break. Surf in places where you feel comfortable and confident.

Be smart. Don't endanger others in the water. If you're riding a wave and other surfers are caught inside of you, be sure to give them enough space. Do not continue on another section of the wave if it will bring you perilously close to other surfers. Even if you technically have the right-of-way, you don't want to risk a collision. If you inadvertently drop in on another surfer who has the right-of-way, cut out of the wave as soon as possible. If someone drops in on a wave in front of you, make a sharp whistling sound to make him or her aware of your presence.

Be generous. Just because you *can* catch every wave doesn't mean you *have* to. Even when the conditions favor stand-up surfers, you shouldn't shut out traditional surfers. Be fair and friendly. Because you have the advantage for spotting set waves, it never hurts to let prone surfers know when a wave is coming.

The experience of surfing is always better when everyone gets along. Do your best as a stand-up surfer to encourage a congenial atmosphere. You can't account for other people's behavior, but your

THE FIVE BASICS OF SURFING ETIQUETTE

1. The first surfer on the wave, or closest to the peak, has the right-of-way.
2. Always paddle around the break to get outside. Surfers on the wave have the right-of-way.
3. Hang on to your board in the impact zone, and look out for other surfers.
4. Help other surfers in trouble.
5. Respect the beach and the ocean.

own actions and attitude can certainly make a difference. Have fun, respect others, and cherish every wave.

Surviving in the Surf

ONE OF THE most overlooked aspects of surfing is paddling outside to the break. This is an essential skill that requires wave knowledge, paddling ability, and endurance. Depending on the beach, getting outside may include negotiating some type of shore break and then pushing through several sections of breaking waves. The size and the strength of the surf will typically determine how difficult it is to get outside. (Reef breaks and some point breaks may have a relatively forgiving channel to paddle through.) No matter what the conditions, your goal should always be to paddle through the impact zone as quickly and efficiently as possible.

Before you get into the water, study the conditions and take note of how often large-set waves are rolling in. Ideally, you want to paddle out directly after a set, so be patient. Before you approach the water, make sure your leash is properly secured to your leg. Walk to the water's edge with your board in one hand and the paddle in the other.

It's often possible, and beneficial, to carry your board beyond the first section of shore break. As you head into the water, keep the board at your side, with the nose facing perpendicular to the incoming surf. Never get between your board and the shore when waves are approaching.

If the surf is small, you may be able to pop up on the board and paddle out in your normal stance. If you find a lot of whitewater and current, it may be easier to paddle in a prone position, with the paddle blade wedged under your chest and the handle facing forward.

A third option is to paddle out on your knees. It's definitely easier to balance this way, but because you have to choke up on the paddle, you lose some of the necessary thrust to push through the surf.

The first rule of paddling through the surf is to paddle hard when the paddling is easy. If you don't see any set waves on the horizon, make a strong effort to get outside of the impact zone. Conversely, if impassable set waves are approaching, it's often best to rest and wait. Paddling out through the break is where you expend most of your energy. Conserving energy in the impact zone will enable you to surf longer and more effectively.

Because of their size, stand-up boards present particular problems in the surf. Unlike smaller surfboards, which can be duck-dived beneath breaking waves, floaty stand-up boards have to be paddled over the top of the wave. Obviously, if you get caught just inside a large section of whitewater, this will be impossible. In this situation, it may be safest to jump off to the side of the board and hang onto it as the wave passes by. If you have time, turn the tail of the board toward the wave and exert downward pressure on the back end, sinking it into the whitewater. Try to keep contact with your board, but never grab the leash or put your finger in the loop of string that secures the leash to the board.

Another method of hanging on to the board is to do what longboard surfers call "turtling." This involves flipping the board over and hanging under water beneath the board, holding the rails as the wave passes overhead. Because of the paddle, this technique is difficult to master with a stand-up board, but with practice you can secure the blade of the paddle between your feet before turtling the board.

If you're far enough away from the breaking waves, you can simply wait out the set. Just sit on the board, straddle it with your legs, and hold the paddle safely away from your face. As the whitewater passes beneath the nose of your board, lean forward and use your free hand to keep the board level. Always keep your feet anchored beneath you to work against being dragged close to shore. Once the set has passed, pop up and paddle quickly to the outside.

Eventually, you'll want to paddle standing up through the surf as much as possible. As you progress, this will get easier, and you'll find yourself capably paddling past sections of whitewater. Most stand-up surfers use a staggered stance when paddling over breaking waves. Use strong, determined strokes as you meet the wave, countering its energy with your own force. If a wave has broken in front of you, shift your weight slightly to your back foot, paddling hard as the whitewater approaches the nose, and then lean forward to level the board as you contact the wave—essentially, you want to push up and over the wave. As the whitewater passes under the board, keep your legs bent and your paddle braced in the water for balance. Then use quick, strong strokes to accelerate past the wave.

Being out in the surf often means dealing with the unexpected. You will get caught inside, and there will be times when you can't hang on to your board. Be safe and proactive at all times. When paddling outside, always give yourself a channel away from other surfers. If you get caught inside and the surf is large, swim your board away from other people in the water—remember that the far end of your board can drag up to 25 feet behind you.

If you know it will be impossible to maintain control of your board, swim toward and beneath the breaking wave. Stay between the board and the wave. As the rush of whitewater passes by and begins to drag you and your board backward, grip your paddle tightly with both hands, holding the blade in front of you and away from your face. The paddle should work as a rudder to bring you to the surface.

Finally, don't panic. Once the wave has passed, use the leash to retrieve the board. If another wave is coming and you can't paddle past it, take a deep breath and repeat the process. Always remain calm, doing your best to conserve energy.

Thriving in the Surf

ONCE YOU'VE MANAGED to paddle outside, the business of catching waves begins. Your next task is to read potential incoming swells and then put yourself in the proper position to catch a wave. As you do this, you need to take several factors into account: the character of the break where you're surfing, the tide, the size of the swell, and the position of other surfers in the water (see the earlier discussion on surf etiquette).

Comprehending these factors, being able to intuit where a wave will break, and then getting yourself in position to catch the wave are skills that are achieved only with time on the water. Beginner surfers should start with smaller, slower breaks, where the waves are more forgiving and the timing and positioning of your takeoff are much less critical.

Ideally, you want to ride on the shoulder of the wave—the sloped section that isn't already breaking. Waves tend to break either left or right. This means that when you're out on the water, the wave you're riding will either be heading toward the beach and to your left (left-breaking) or toward the beach and to your right (right-breaking). Depending on the break, each individual wave may be predominantly left-breaking, predominantly right-breaking, or capable of being ridden left and right. Point breaks and reef breaks will typically be clearly defined as lefts and rights, as opposed to beach breaks, where the direction may change according to the swell and the tide.

As a swell approaches, look for the peak of the wave. The best point at which to take off on a wave is on the section of the shoulder closest to the peak—either to the left or the right of the peak, depending on the direction of the break. This is when you need to be proactive. Without heading too far outside, paddle aggressively toward the predominant shoulder, and then bring the nose of your board about until it's facing the direction in which the wave is breaking, that is, the direction in which you want to ride.

Knowing how to perform a pivot turn is beneficial. Not only will you be able to rotate your board faster, but utilizing the pivot turn puts you in a staggered surf-stance as the wave approaches. Many beginners tend to turn their board too early and then wait for the wave to arrive behind them. The problem with this technique is that you can't see the wave as it approaches from behind, which may result in several surprises: The wave may break behind you or be steeper than you anticipated, or there may even already be another unseen surfer on the wave (someone who paddled aggressively toward the peak and pivoted onto the wave). Do your best to maintain eye contact with the wave, paddling hard to position your board and turning at the last opportune moment.

Once you've turned onto a wave, paddle in short, quick strokes to gain momentum and catch the wave. Depending on the size, strength, and steepness of the wave, the amount of paddling you'll have to do will vary greatly. Again, this is why it's important to take off near the peak; the farther out you are on the shoulder, the more difficult it will be to catch the wave.

Ideally, after taking a few quick strokes on one side of the board, the energy of the wave will thrust you forward. If you have to paddle numerous strokes to catch the wave, then the board may start to turn, which may force you to switch sides with the paddle. Unfortunately, this can be a momentum-killer. Try to position yourself so the board will be facing in the proper direction when you catch the wave. Anticipate which way the board will be turning, and adjust the angle of your approach to accommodate. If you still find yourself turning too far away from the shoulder, keep the paddle blade close to, or even underneath, the rail of the board, paddling energetically to get on the wave. If this fails and you do have to switch hands, you'll have to make the transition quickly—once you lose momentum, you miss the wave.

Pitfalls (or Success)

THREE THINGS CAN happen when you are paddling for a wave, and two of them are bad:

1. **You don't catch the wave.** This could be because you were too far out on the shoulder (away from the peak), you were too far outside, or you didn't paddle hard enough or effectively enough to get the wave. Expect this to happen several times as you begin to surf, or as you get acquainted with a new spot. Learning to read the waves and effectively position the board takes time. Beyond skill, you need confidence and determination. Again, be proactive: Paddle aggressively to position yourself near the peak, then use strong, even strokes to catch the wave.
2. **The wave breaks behind you or is too steep to catch when you start paddling for it.** This is also a by-product of inexperience. As you learn to pivot the board quickly, you'll be able to keep the wave in view as you approach an open spot on the shoulder. This will enable you to better position yourself and avoid getting run over by the wave.
3. **You successfully catch the wave.** In this case, read on.

Riding the Wave

THERE WILL LIKELY be plenty of times when you think you've caught a wave, but then you don't and the wave passes by. But when you do catch one, you'll know: The momentum of the swell will accelerate you forward, and you'll feel the board gliding beneath you. At this point, if your feet are still parallel, you should step back into your surf stance. (I assume everyone knows if they are regular-footed or goofy-footed, but just for clarification: Regular foot means left foot forward and right foot back, and goofy foot means right foot forward and left foot back.)

As the board thrusts forward and then becomes propelled by the energy of the wave, bend your knees and maintain a balanced position between your front and back leg.

Here are three more potential pitfalls and how to prevent them:

1. **When the wave thrusts the board forward, you lose your balance and fall off the back of the board.** Always keep enough pressure in your front foot, but not too much.
2. **Your board "pearls" as you head down the face of the wave.** This is when the nose of your board goes under water and ejects you from the board. Pearling typically happens if you don't have your rear foot back far enough or you can't get it back quickly enough. Also, on steep waves you may need ride to down the wave face at an angle—the steeper the wave, the sharper the angle. Remember: *Your board is big.*

3. **You glide straight out in front of the wave and can't stay on the shoulder.** As you ride down the face of a wave, you need to set yourself up for a bottom turn (see below). On smaller and slower waves, this may be just a subtle redirection of the board, but faster and steeper waves often require aggressive action to keep the board on course.

Frontside Versus Backside

MOST BEGINNING STAND-UP surfers will prefer to ride frontside on a wave. For a regular-footer, this means going right on the wave; for a goofy-footer, it means going left. Of course, the wave pretty much dictates the direction in which you'll surf. Eventually, though, you'll want to learn to ride waves both frontside and backside. SUP boards can be a bit cumbersome to ride backside, but not only can it definitely be done, there are many stand-up surfers who excel at it.

The Bottom Turn

AN ESSENTIAL TOOL for advanced wave-riding, a bottom turn provides one of the best sensations in all of surfing—stepping on the inside rail of your board and carving back up the face of the wave. A proper bottom turn will propel you down the line of the wave and set you up for advanced surfing maneuvers like off-the-lips and cutbacks.

As you drop down the face of the wave, your rear foot should be positioned over your board's back fin(s). When you reach the bottom of the wave, initiate the turn by applying pressure to your rear foot. (Waiting until you reach the relatively flat section of the wave will allow your fins to grip better through the turn.) Use your paddle as a pivot point, dragging it slightly behind you and along the wave face to help activate the turn. Bracing with the paddle will also help you maintain your balance as you lean into the wave.

Because SUP boards are wide, it will help to move your back foot to the inside rail of the board. If you are riding frontside and turning toeside, the ball of your foot should be as close to the inside rail as possible, and just over the fin. If you're riding backside, you should position your heel just above the inside rail to initiate the turn, bracing the paddle behind you for balance.

Once you master the technique, you should be able to turn most SUP boards. With larger boards, you may find it necessary to apply strong pressure on the rear foot, stomping on the inside rail, to get the board to turn.

Smaller boards definitely turn quicker and more effectively. Boards with displacement hulls or thick, rounded rails aren't good for executing bottom turns (however, these boards aren't typically recommended for down-the-line surfing).

Maximizing Your Experience

ONCE YOU'VE NAILED your bottom turn and you're heading back up the face of the wave, you're ready to perform a top turn. Essentially, you need to reverse the action of the bottom turn, switching your rear foot to the opposite rail and applying pressure to carve back down the face of the wave. If the section of the wave is steep, you should maintain pressure on the back foot to keep from pearling the board. Once you've made it down the face of the wave, you can set up for another bottom turn.

As you carve turns on the wave, you'll need to switch your rear foot from rail to rail, alternating pressure from one side to the other. Use your paddle as a tool, flaring it into the wave face to help you initiate turns and using it as a brace to help you maintain your balance. Staying in the critical section of the wave and maintaining board speed will allow for more effective and satisfying turns.

Every wave is different and must be ridden according to its own characteristics. Slow, gentle waves won't allow you to carve dramatic turns, but these waves are appropriate for beginners since they come with fewer critical consequences and allow the surfer more reaction time. Faster, steeper waves offer more thrill but also require more skill.

Always pay attention to where you are on the wave and what the wave is doing. If you get too far out on the shoulder, away from the critical breaking section, the wave may pass you by. Sometimes it's necessary to reverse direction or cut back on a wave, finding a relatively steeper section of the face, in order to maintain momentum and board speed. Conversely, if a wave is closing out and about to break on you, you must often turn straight on the wave and outrun the whitewater.

Another option is to cut out of the wave and start paddling back to the break. Many beginning surfers are reluctant to cut out of the wave, feeling they're sacrificing riding time, but cutting out of waves is often a smart strategy that allows you to avoid getting caught inside, therefore saving you the energy to catch more waves.

If the wave is breaking too fast and you can't cut out of the wave, it sometimes helps to turn out in front of the whitewater and then, as soon as it's safe, dive off the board and duck under the pursuing wave. You'll have to retrieve your board (via the leash) to start paddling out again, but at least you won't have to paddle all the way from the beach.

Wiping Out

IT'S GOING TO happen, and when it does, you need to be (there's that word again) proactive. If a wave knocks you down, try to maintain control of the board. Ideally, you don't want it to squirt away from you and potentially hit other surfers. When the wave is too large or the situation too critical, you need to protect yourself. If you lose control of the board, try to distance yourself from the board, jumping away and in the direction opposite the one in which the board is traveling. If the wave is sending the board toward you, dive beneath the surface of the water. If you're not sure what's happening, use your free arm to protect your head.

Most of these reactions come naturally. Above all else, remain calm. Don't panic, and don't forget to breathe before you go under.

As a beginner, you are going to fall. As you progress and take on more-challenging conditions, you will fall some more. This is all part of the process; getting frustrated will not make you a better stand-up surfer. Have fun, surf smart, and be safe.

A SoCal SUS Sampler

THE FOLLOWING CHAPTER details popular stand-up-surfing spots in Southern California. Of course, this isn't a comprehensive list: Depending on the swell and season, there are plenty of additional breaks along the coast—both heralded and unheralded—that are ideal for surfing on a paddleboard.

As with "Paddling the Southland" (page 43), the geographic regions are arranged from south to north and separated by county. Some of the previous destinations that contain information about surfing have also been cross-referenced here.

Dropping in near La Jolla Shores (see page 163)

Photo courtesy of Izzy Tihanyi/Surf Diva

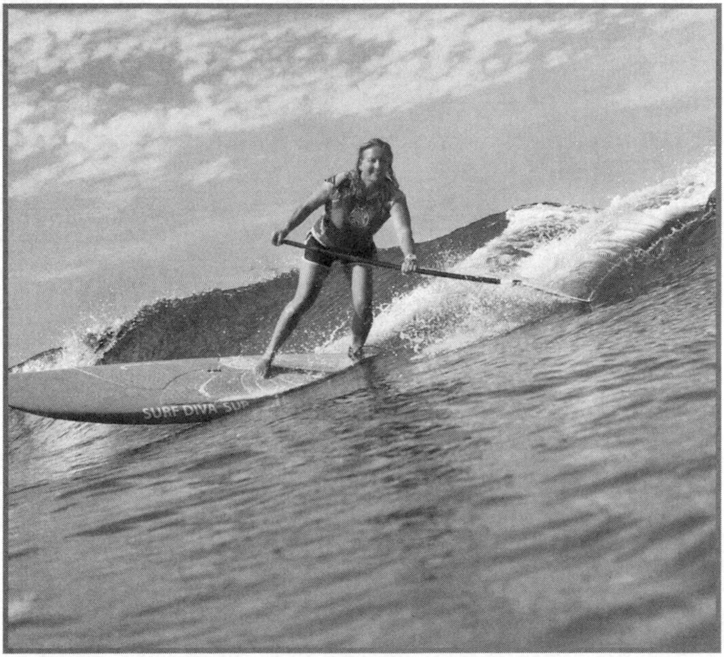

San Diego County

Tourmaline Surfing Park

San Diego

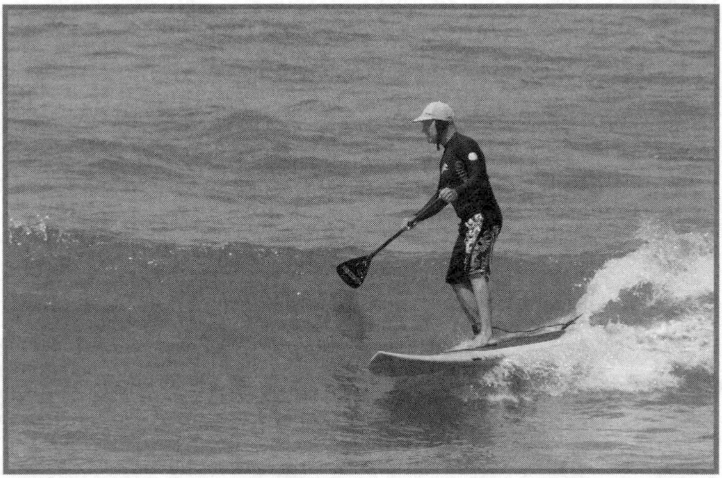

Catching a small one on a nice summer day

Overview Head down to the parking lot at the end of Tourmaline Street, and the first thing you'll notice are the vans—lots of them, all with boards strapped on top or tucked inside. Along with the vans are a crew of locals who look like they've been coming to this beach, hanging ten and just hanging out, every day for the last 30 years. And they have.

Tourmaline Surfing Park is that kind of place. Like San Onofre or Waikiki Beach, "Tourmo" is a legendary surf spot, known as much for its history and social aspects as for its waves. Stand-up surfers first started coming here in 2006, and while they still seem to be a small part of the scene, they have become a consistent part of it.

Unlike San Onofre or Doheny Beach (see pages 169–183), Tourmaline has no boundaries for stand-up surfing. That can be good

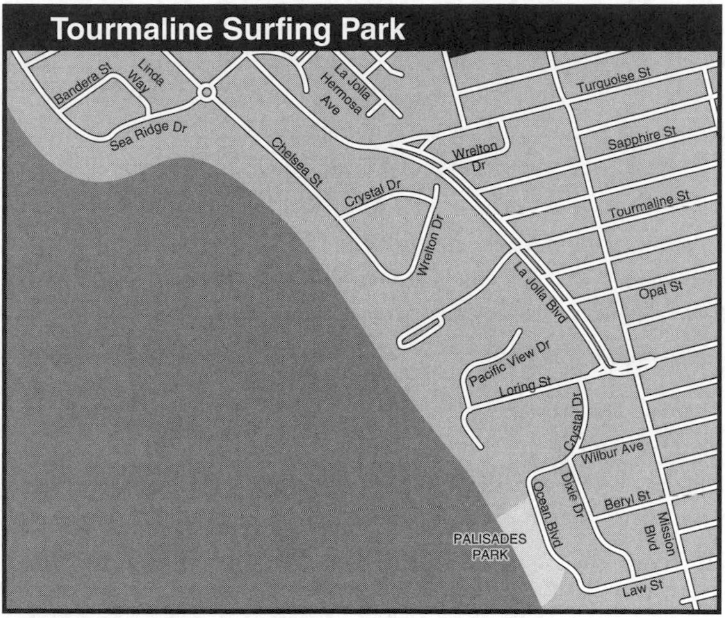

and bad. Stand-up surfers have access to all the breaks, but they also have to contend with tight crowds of prone surfers. It's definitely a forgiving wave, and on most days it's ideal for those learning to stand-up surf, but crowds are an issue. For someone without any type of surfing experience, the concentration of boards in the lineup will be intimidating. Many of the local stand-up surfers advise those new to Tourmaline to paddle out early in the morning, before the zoo factor sets in. For those still working on their surfing skills, I would also advise avoiding concentrations of prone surfers and finding a less-populated section of the beach to catch waves. As always, show respect for the local crew of prone surfers who've been coming to Tourmaline for many years.

Where to Surf There are several places to line up at Tourmaline, but not every break will work in every swell. The best-known and most consistent breaks are **Pumphouse** (south of the parking lot), **Tourmaline** (directly in front of the parking lot), and **Old Man's** (just to the north).

Pumphouse forms off a sandbar and peaks left and right. Tourmaline breaks right and then terminates in a small channel (perfect for paddling out). Old Man's is—you guessed it—a slow reef break. All the breaks are generally of the slower longboard variety.

Like many breaks in the San Diego area, Tourmo has consistent waves throughout most of the year. Winter swells from the west and northwest will have the most energy. South swells may be better at breaks farther north, but that doesn't dissuade the crew of Tourmaline regulars. In the summer months, the scene really comes together here—good times with warm water, sunshine, and a few fun waves.

Directions and Parking Tourmaline Street intersects La Jolla Boulevard about 2.5 miles south of downtown La Jolla. Head west down the hill until you reach the parking lot. Parking is free. There are probably about 100 spaces in the lot, but this is a popular beach, so it will fill up. There is also some additional street parking on Tourmaline Street above the lot.

Ability Level Not recommended for beginners because of the crowds. For anyone new to the beach, I would suggest arriving early and maybe gaining advice (or at least well-wishes) from someone in the local crew of stand-up surfers. Many of the prone surfers have been coming here since the Bronze Age, so try to show them a bit of deference.

Tide Low to medium works best.

Swell Direction Northwest, west, and southwest are the favored directions.

Facilities Outdoor showers and restrooms. At the end of the parking lot, there's a nice viewing area for watching the surf and the scene.

Water Quality San Diego fares better than Orange or Los Angeles County in the water-quality department, but Tourmaline is one of the more polluted beaches in San Diego County. As at all beaches, exercise caution after winter storms.

Conditions and Hazards Perhaps getting hit by a 12-foot longboard. Otherwise, the break seems safe and friendly. At low tide, your fin might find a submerged rock to the north of Old Man's.

Special Note Tourmaline was dedicated as a surf park in 1963—the first facility of its kind in the country.

Local Burrito Taco Surf Taco Shop (4657 Mission Blvd.; 858-272-3877, **tacosurftacoshop.com**): See Mission Bay, page 53, for details.

La Jolla Shores San Diego

(See map on page 55)

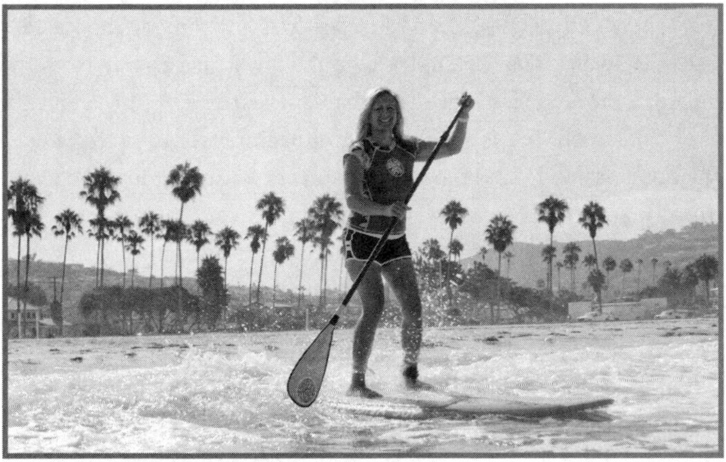

Paddling through the breakwater near La Jolla

Photo courtesy of Izzy Tihanyi/Surf Diva

Overview La Jolla is famous for its touristy beaches and scenic vistas. And while it will never be known as a surfing destination, it does have waves—sometimes huge ones. Depending on conditions, La Jolla Shores can be ideal for both beginner and experienced stand-up surfers.

Where to Surf For those unfamiliar with the area, it helps to know the lay of the land. The best strategy, as in many locales, is to avoid conflict with prone surfers. To this end, steer clear of the area near **Scripps Pier**—the fast beach break here is often packed with shortboarders. A better option for stand-up surfers is to access the beach at **The Marine Room** restaurant (see the SUP chapter on La Jolla, page 54, for details) and head south. The break is between the launch spot and the La Jolla cliffs. On any decent west swell, there should be other paddle surfers. The wave jacks up as it passes over a series of outside reefs before reforming and sectioning on the inside. It's a fun SUP wave when it's working. In the winter this wave, and particularly the wave farther out on the point, can be quite large, so use caution when heading out.

If you don't find any surf to the south of The Marine Room, there may still be some small fun sections in front of the **La Jolla Beach & Tennis Club.** Again, try to stake out a space away from the lineup of prone surfers. If you're unsure, head north to the vicinity of the boat launch. This is an ideal spot for beginners—the wave is slow, the beach is sandy, and most prone surfers want nothing to do with the kayakers (there is still plenty of room to avoid them). The key, as always, is to be aware of the conditions and your surroundings. La Jolla Shores is a beautiful place, and any day on the water here, particularly one when you're catching waves, is pretty great.

Directions and Parking Exit I-5 at La Jolla Village Drive. Head west on La Jolla Village for 0.7 mile, then turn left on Torrey Pines Road. After 2.2 miles, turn right onto Little Street. Follow Little Street as it veers left, then take the first right onto St. Louis Terrace. After 0.1 mile, turn right on Spindrift Drive and look for parking. The Marine Room (2000 Spindrift Drive) will be straight ahead on the left. The beach access is on the south side of the restaurant.

Conditions and Hazards The breaks work best on west swells. In the summer months, the waves will tend to be smaller and beginner-friendly. In the winter, the surf can be large. In fact, the point outside La Jolla Cove will occasionally produce massive waves in the 20-foot range.

Unless the surf is large, you have few hazards to worry about beyond lurking stingrays. Be sure to shuffle your feet when entering and exiting the water.

Restrictions The breaks are pretty much self-policed, but lifeguards will probably keep stand-up surfers away from the concentration of swimmers. In summertime, this will definitely include the shoreline in front of La Jolla Shores Park.

Lessons and Rentals **Surf Diva** (2160 Avenida de la Playa; 858-454-8273, **surfdiva.com**): See the SUP profile of La Jolla, page 58, for details.

Cardiff Reef Encinitas

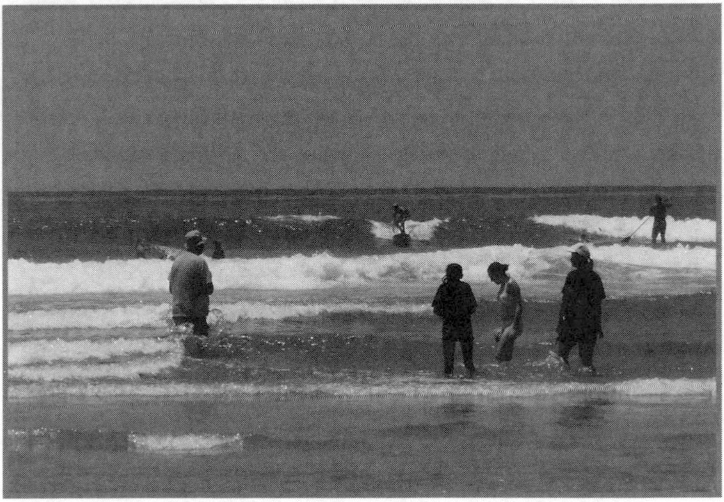

Surf breaks south of the La Jolla Beach and Tennis Club.

Overview Just north of Solana Beach, where the San Elijo River feeds into the ocean, one finds the fun and consistent surf break at Cardiff Reef, in San Elijo State Park. With easy access from the highway, a decent amount of beachfront parking (it's a state park, so payment or an annual pass is required), and a nearby campground, the spot is a popular destination for all types of surfers. On warm summer days,

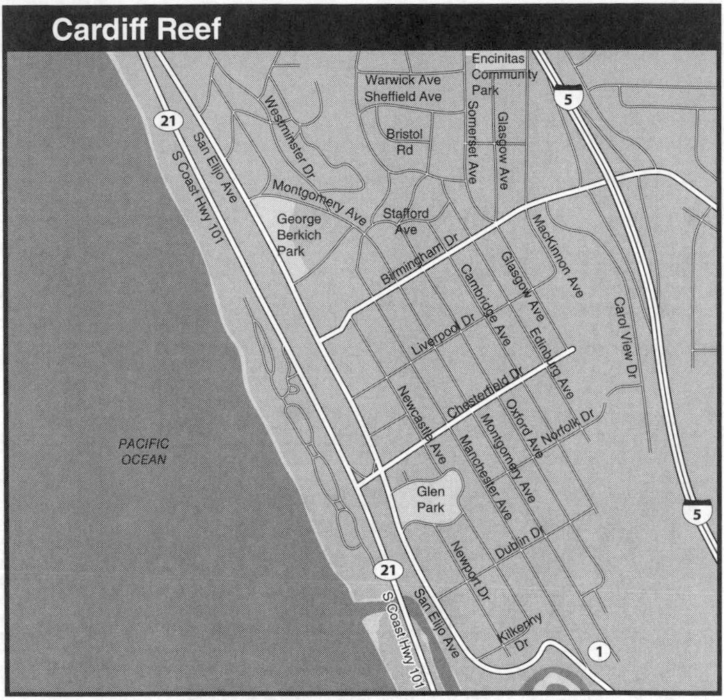

entire families of surfers flock here, sharing the water with the local shortboard, longboard, and stand-up surfers. The last group is the newest addition to the lineup, but perhaps the most consistent and enthusiastic.

Over the past few years, Cardiff Reef has become the most popular and established stand-up surfing spot in north San Diego County. (Because of its proximity to **San Elijo State Beach Campground,** Cardiff is also a fun weekend getaway spot.) Unlike other state parks, San Elijo has no restrictions on where SUPers can launch or ride waves, but stand-up surfers should pay particular attention to the crowd of younger and less experienced surfers, particularly when paddling or riding close to shore.

Where to Surf Launching here is quite easy because of the foot-friendly sandbars that form around the river mouth. The underwater reefs are about 50 yards offshore. The wave is generally a peaky, rolling right-hander that first breaks across a series of flat, grass-covered rocks, then backs off, and then re-forms inside over the shifting sandbars formed by the river. In the summer, the break is typically a fairly mushy longboard-style wave—not too fast, not too large, and generally easy to paddle out to, but during large winter swells, the wave transforms into a roaring right-hand point break. On these days, the paddle out can be difficult, but for the experienced, the reward level is quite high.

If crowds at Cardiff Reef become prohibitive, stand-up surfers might also want to try the SUP-friendly wave at **Table Rock.** To get there, head about south of the campground toward the main drag of Solana Beach, then park at the beachside lot at the south end of San Elijo Lagoon. The break, which is about 100 yards offshore, should be less crowded than the main break at Cardiff, but it's also more fickle, needing less tide and more swell than Cardiff Reef. For goofy-footers, there is a left-hand break known as **Suckouts** about 50 yards north of the main peak at Cardiff Reef. It's a single peak that works best at low tide. Note, however, that the takeoff zone is fairly narrow, and Suckouts becomes quickly crowded. Trying to stand-up-surf this section might be challenging—and probably not recommended—if there is already a crew of prone surfers lined up at the peak.

Directions and Parking Cardiff Reef lies within San Elijo State Park. From I-5, exit at Birmingham Drive. Head west on Birmingham, continue 0.5 mile, and then turn left on San Elijo Avenue. Take the first right onto Chesterfield Drive and then a quick left onto South Coast Highway 101. The state park day-use entrance is about 0.4 mile away on the right. The state park lot offers a decent amount of beachfront parking. For those who don't have a pass, payment can be made at the kiosks in the parking lot ($10 per day; annual passes run $195). It's just a short walk from the parking lot to the water. Free parking is available on Highway 101 on either side of the campground entrance.

Facilities Beachfront parking, outdoor showers, and restrooms. Camping is available at San Elijo State Beach Campground.

Ability Level On normal days, Cardiff will appeal to people of all ages and abilities. When the surf gets large, the wave gains speed and strength, and the paddle out can be difficult. There is a fairly regular crew of stand-up surfers at the break, which should be reassuring for beginners.

Break Direction The main break is a right. Suckouts breaks left just north of the mouth of the San Elijo River.

Crowds Moderate to crowded. Expect to see families of beginning surfers on the inside portion of the break.

Tide Low to medium works best.

Swell Direction This is a very consistent wave capable of working in most swell directions. Large winter swells will provide the most punch.

Water Quality The reef's proximity to San Elijo Lagoon is a significant problem in the winter. Those who don't want a trip to the ENT doctor should avoid surfing here after any significant rainstorm.

Local burrito My friend Ken, the burrito aficionado, complains about how carne asada burritos in Orange County, for some unknown reason, don't come with guacamole. Ken spent many years in San Diego, where, he claims, all carne asada burritos come with guacamole. Apparently there is a line in the sand between San Diego and Orange Counties where the avocados stop flowing. For those traveling from the DGZ (de-guacamolized zone), and for anyone wanting a post-surf burrito, **Roberto's** in Solana Beach is a nice option (445 N. Highway 101; 858-704-4075). Besides the carne asada, they have plenty of other choices, including the humongous Lifeguard Burrito, recommended for two people and guaranteed to keep you out of the water for at least an hour.

Orange County

San Onofre State Beach: Trails

Near San Clemente

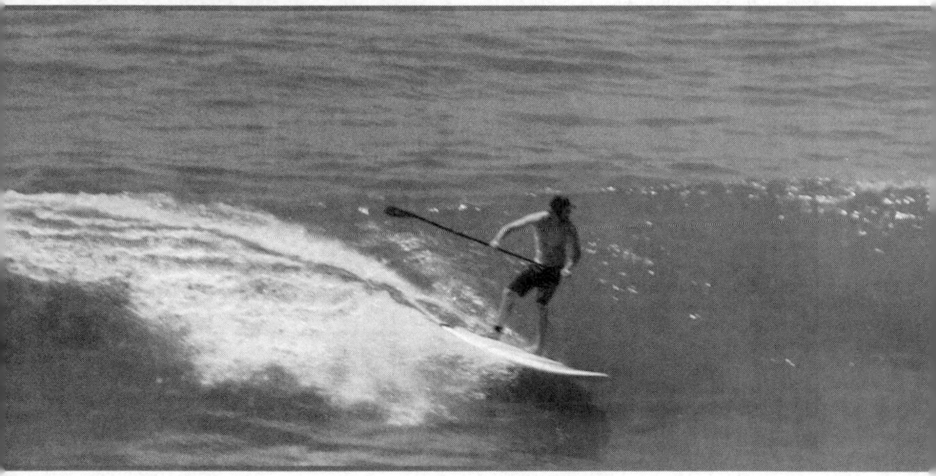

More surfing action at Trails

Overview At the south end of San Onofre State Park, adjacent to the hills of Camp Pendleton, lies a series of beach breaks known simply as Trails. To get there, bypass the primary entrance to San Onofre, continue past the voluptuous twin domes of the nuclear power plant, and enter the park at the south gate. A bluffside road parallels the shore for roughly 3 miles, and beach access comes via six numbered trails. Look for one of the specific trailhead signs, park in the adjacent day-use lot, and then be prepared for a hike (for the stand-up paddler, I recommend using a carrying strap). The beach trails are wide and graded, but each courses down a rather significant bluff.

Although the hike at Trails can be a bit taxing (particularly the trip back up the bluff after a long surf session), it also can be quite

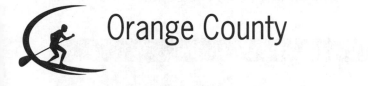

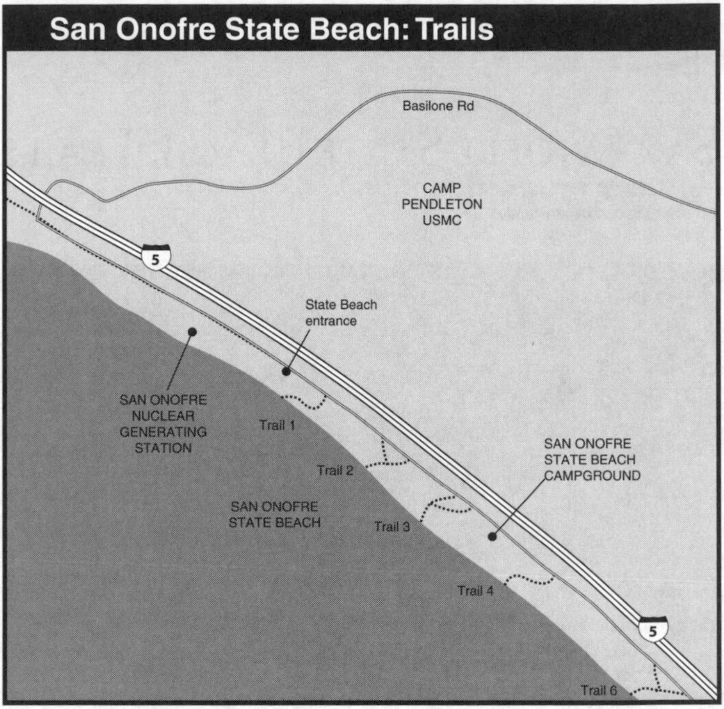

rewarding. Every trip to these beaches promises an air of adventure. The coastal bluffs are beautiful—dramatically eroded and laden with coastal sage—and the views of the ocean, the sandstone cliffs, and the uncrowded beaches may remind one of northern Baja California (if northern Baja had a nuclear power plant). A trip to Dog Patch at San Onofre may be easier and more convenient, but a trip to Trails offers an opportunity to get away from the crowds and explore any number of uncrowded peaks. Some days there will be more than a hundred surfers out at San Onofre but only handful at Trail 1. (Of course, this quotient changes when a line forms at the main entrance to San Onofre. On those days, there are more surfers willing to make the pilgrimage to Trails.)

Where to Surf Because it encompasses roughly 3 miles of coastline, Trails offers a great variety of surfing conditions. On a given day, it's not uncommon to find shortboarders, longboarders, bodyboarders, and stand-up surfers all working adjacent peaks. Although Trails is essentially a series of beach breaks, outside sandbars and reefs allow for long, workable shoulders in the right conditions. The break at any particular spot can vary dramatically based on tide height and swell direction. The key to surfing Trails is to find a spot or a peak that is working at the moment. The conditions can be fickle, so always check a particular break before going out.

Trail 1 has a lookout with views of the waves at the foot of this trail and Trail 2. When sussing out the break, be sure to take into account the tide height and the distance the waves are breaking from shore (typically the farther out, the better). Trail 1 has three major breaks and may consistently have the best shape in winter, but it's also the most crowded. Although there is rarely competitive vibe at any of the trails, **Trails 2 and 3** may be better options for less-proficient stand-up surfers because there will be fewer, if any, boarders to avoid and fewer watchful eyes. A surf camp operates out of **Trail 4,** where the waves tend to be slow and mushy. During summer south swells, when the upper trails tend to get walled, **Trail 6** becomes a popular option.

Because the tall cliffs intensify the wind, all of the breaks along Trails are subject to getting blown out. Even on days when there are perfect offshore winds at San Onofre proper, there can be chopped-up side-shore winds at Trails. Again, make the trip to the bluff and check the surf before going out.

Just like Dogpatch and Doheny, Trails is chock-full of foot-bruising stones along the shore. If you go out at low tide, either wear booties or look for a sandy stretch of foot-friendly shore access. Unlike Dogpatch and Doheny, Trails can be difficult and challenging when it comes to paddling out through the surf. Because of the shifting nature of the peaks, there is rarely a perfect channel for paddling. On large-surf days, the task of getting outside can be difficult and even exhausting. Always pay attention to the duration, the size, and the consistency of the set waves. If you get caught inside, it may be better to wait out a set before paddling out.

Once you make it outside, it may behoove you to not ride the waves all the way inside—one additional carve-toward-shore turn may result in an extra 10 minutes of effort to get back outside the break. Once you're in the lineup, keep an eye out for outside waves. More than other local breaks, Trails seems to have an ability to produce some unexpected outside peaks. For the well-prepared, these waves are capable of providing long, memorable rides as they bowl up and then re-form toward the beach. For the ill-prepared, outside waves will merely result in more frustrating dives under the rolling whitewater.

No discussion of Trails is complete without mentioning sharks. In 2003 a whale beached, died, and was covered in sand along this stretch. Unfortunately, whale oil leached into the water and attracted predators. There were plenty of shark sightings that year, and Trails gained a reputation as a haven for great white sharks.

A decade later, the dead whale's remnants are long gone, but the reputation persists. Of course, it's not entirely undeserved. When researchers want to track juvenile great white sharks, they search in two places along the California coast: at the point where Sunset Boulevard meets Pacific Coast Highway in Malibu and in front of the San Onofre nuclear power plant. The shark researchers know their subject—plenty of juvenile great whites frequent the waters around San Onofre. What the shark researchers also know, however, is that juvenile great white sharks don't attack humans. Because they're juveniles, they typically measure less than 9 feet long. This seems pretty substantial, but it isn't really by great white shark standards. Talk to any longtime surfer at Trails, and they probably have at least one story about sighting a shark.

So should you be concerned about sharks? Probably not. Although being eaten seems particularly heinous and scary, it's very unlikely. Worry about driving on the freeway instead. Your chances of being attacked by a shark are more remote than winning the lottery. If you see a fin in the water, it's most likely a dolphin. You'll know if you watch: Dolphins are graceful in the water and jump into

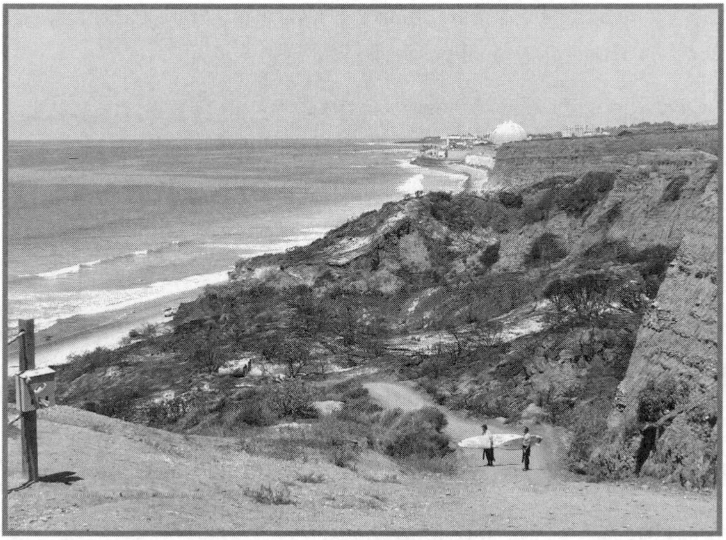

Looking down from Trail 1. The nuclear power plant is in the distance, and Dog Patch is just beyond that.

the air with poise and aplomb. If a shark jumps out of the water, it looks crazed, out of its element, and none too happy. They don't jump in a graceful scalloping motion; they come out shivering and shaking, engaging in some sort of prehistoric flop. The sharks are out there—they always have been—but it's best not to think about them.

Update, spring 2015: There have been a slew of shark sightings at Trail 1. I've seen several myself, mostly juveniles in the 5- to 6-foot range. Most surfers seem unfazed by this development. The sharks seem to mostly mind their own business, feeding on bait fish and small stingrays.

Directions and Parking From I-5, exit at Basilone Road and head south, past the main state park entrance and the power plant, until you reach the south entrance of the park. Parking for Trail 1 is about 300 yards past the south entrance. The other trails are farther down the road. Parking is typically available at every trail. For day use, though, be sure not to park in the camping areas.

Trails is part of San Onofre, a California State Park. Day use costs $15, and an annual pass is $195.

Hazards Lots of small stones along the shore. Impact on the feet varies significantly with the tides.

See my notes above about sharks. While no one has been attacked here and the sharks tend to be relatively small (and most likely not dangerous), it never hurts to keep an eye on the water.

Facilities There are outdoor showers and no-frills restrooms near each trailhead.

Ability Level The sparse crowds are advantageous for beginners, but depending on surf size, the conditions can be intermediate to advanced. The paddle out can be challenging during large swell events.

Break Direction Peaky, both lefts and rights.

Crowds Generally light—the best thing about Trails. Long-period winter swells will see Trail 1 get a bit crowded. Trail 6 attracts a substantial crowd of longboarders on summer weekends.

Tides Depends on the trail, but generally low to medium is best.

Best Swell Direction Winter swells and spring-wind swells work at Trails 1–3. In the summer, when south swells wall up at Trail 1, Trail 6 might be a better option. Combo swells will help with the shape.

Rules Stand-up surfers are allowed at Trails. On crowded weekends, it might be best to stay clear of some of the more congested breaks.

Water Quality No urban runoff near Trails, but the porous cliffs may dirty the water after large rainstorms.

San Onofre State Beach: Dog Patch **Near San Clemente**

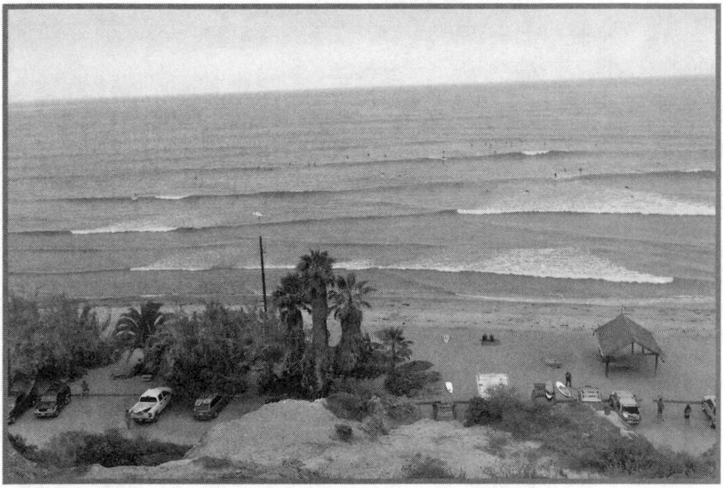

An overview of the breaks at San Onofre. Dog Patch is on the left side of the frame.

Overview Few places have greater standing in the annals of California surfing than San Onofre. Surfers first came here in the wake of World War II armed with thick balsa boards and a desire to ride the slow, peeling waves. San Onofre quickly became the Waikiki of Southern California—not a mere testing ground for the sport, but a place that came to be the very embodiment of the surfing lifestyle. Pioneering watermen spent their summers here diving for abalone, building bonfires, and camping on the beach. Who wouldn't want to be a part of that? It's easy to see how the sport of surfing grew in popularity and later spawned a cultural phenomenon. Its practitioners were fit, tan, and, beyond riding waves, without a care in the world.

Seventy years later, the surfing culture still thrives at San Onofre. Surfers of all types flock here to ride the consistently rolling waves. On weekends—or just about any sunny day—the long stretch

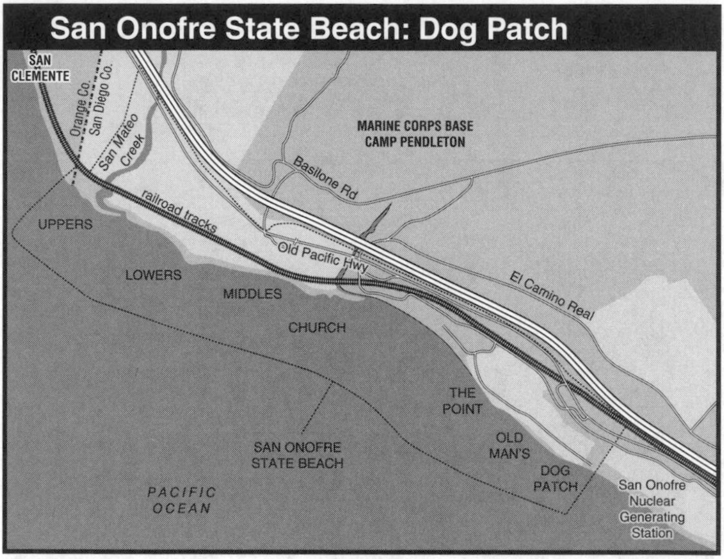

of beachfront parking is full of cars, trucks, and surf vans. A core group of surf dudes seems to be here every day. They're easily spotted because they are such perfect caricatures of what it means to be an aging surfer—guys whose names should be Duke, Moondoggie, or the Big Kahuna. Of course, if you talk to them for a few minutes, you'll find out that their names actually *are* Duke, Moondoggie, and the Big Kahuna. San Onofre is that kind of place.

Where to Surf Although the surfing tends to be more social than serious, San Onofre can produce some fun peeling shoulders. What the waves lack in punch, they make up for with length and consistency. The wave breaks pretty much year-round, in all types of swells; however, the best waves are found during south swells. Of the three breaks here, the first two being **The Point** and **Old Man's,** only the southernmost, **Dog Patch,** is open to stand-up surfers. When entering the park, continue driving past the long line of parked cars to the vicinity of the volleyball courts. On the bluff south of Old Man's are two black poles—one with an O sign and the other with a K sign.

Stand-up surfers must stay to the south of this pair of signs. When in the water, the signs should read OK. If you venture out of the legal stand-up zone, the OK message transforms—those state park folks are clever—to a less inviting KO. If this seems difficult to interpret (or if you suffer from myopia), don't fret—there's always a crew of stand-up surfers at Dog Patch. You'll find plenty of folks in the water and on the beach to provide information about the boundaries.

Crowds are an issue at Dogpatch, but the scene is typically friendly and congenial. For the most part, the prone surfers stick at Old Man's and The Point, leaving Dog Patch to the stand-up surfers. Staying within the legal boundary means there's no chance of being harassed.

On good surf days, Dog Patch has multiple peaks, which help accommodate the crowds. The wave tends to roll in slowly, cresting over soft-mounded reefs, then backing and re-forming before breaking slowly to the beach. It's a user-friendly wave that appeals to a wide range of skill levels—fun and accessible for beginners, but wide open and section-y enough to appeal to those wanting to improve their skills or try new maneuvers.

When the surf is good here, expect to find a core group of accomplished stand-up surfers deftly showing off their abilities. On large swells and lower tides, there is an additional break offshore of the nuclear power plant. Known as **Nukes** (go figure), the wave can be a good alternative to Dog Patch. It's a longer paddle to reach the break, but Nukes tends to be less crowded.

Directions and Parking From I-5, exit at Basilone Road and head south for 1.3 miles. Turn right onto Beach Club Road, toward the main entrance to the state park. Continue right, away from the nuclear plant, and toward the entrance kiosk. (On busy days, you may find a queue to get in the park. If this is the case, follow the signs to the dirt lot to the left of the kiosk.) Past the entrance, continue down the hill and onto the dirt road that runs parallel to the beach. Keep heading south. The stand-up-surfing area is at the far end of the parking lot. Day use is $15, and an annual pass costs $195.

Hazards Lots of small stones along the shore. Surf booties may be required for the tenderfooted.

Facilities Outdoor showers are strategically placed in small groves of bamboo. There are also changing rooms and restrooms. The beach has volleyball courts, fire pits, and picnic tables. People come here to surf, and then they stay to socialize, picnic, and barbecue.

Ability Level The user-friendly wave should be fine for beginners on most days. Experienced riders will enjoy maneuvering through the sections, using the wave to push their skill levels.

Crowds Definitely a factor, but not a deal-breaker. There are always a lot of folks on the water, but they tend to be friendly.

Tides Medium is best. Too low and you'll have a long course of cobblestones to navigate before getting to the water; too high and the wave tends to break close to shore. Of course, bigger swells will handle higher tides.

Best Swell Direction San Onofre picks up all swell directions. South swells may be the best.

Rules Stand-up surfers are required to stay south of the OK marker.

Water Quality The water tends to be clean here. The obvious exception is after large rainstorms, when runoff from the cliffs and San Juan Creek mucks up the near-shore waters.

Doheny State Beach

Dana Point

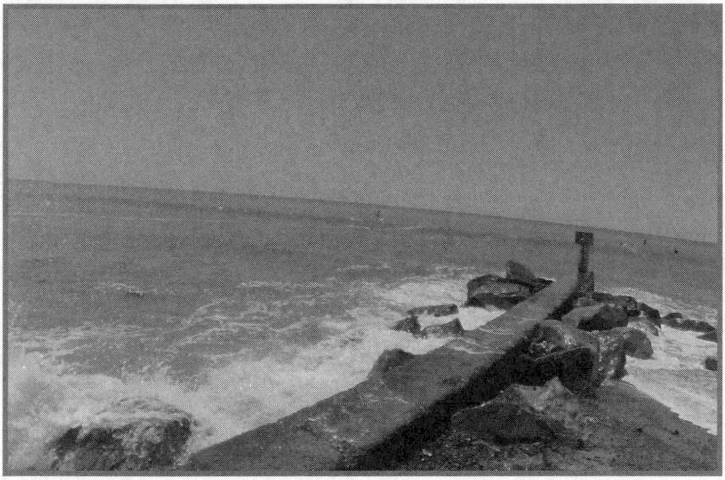

Thor's Hammer at Doheny State Beach

Overview Just south of Dana Point Harbor, nestled between the protruding rock breakwater and the long strand of Capistrano Beach, one finds Doheny State Beach. Its 300 yards of shallow reefs and rocky shoreline compose a fabled longboard surf break, made famous in the 1960s by the likes of The Beach Boys and The Surfaris. The latter group's "Surfer Joe" spent his days here before he was shipped off to Camp Pendleton, and through the years, legions of less-legendary surfers have made Doheny their home as well.

On summer days, the break is littered with beginning surfers; kid surfers; packs of old, wily longboarders; and, in recent years, a burgeoning crew of stand-up surfers. Every one of these groups is there for the same reason—Doheny is the one of the easiest, friendliest, and most accessible waves in Southern California.

My first time stand-up surfing at Doheny, on a Friday afternoon in late September, left much to be desired. What I didn't know, however, is that I had chosen the weekend of the **Battle of the Paddle** for my maiden outing. This racing event attracts top pro and amateur

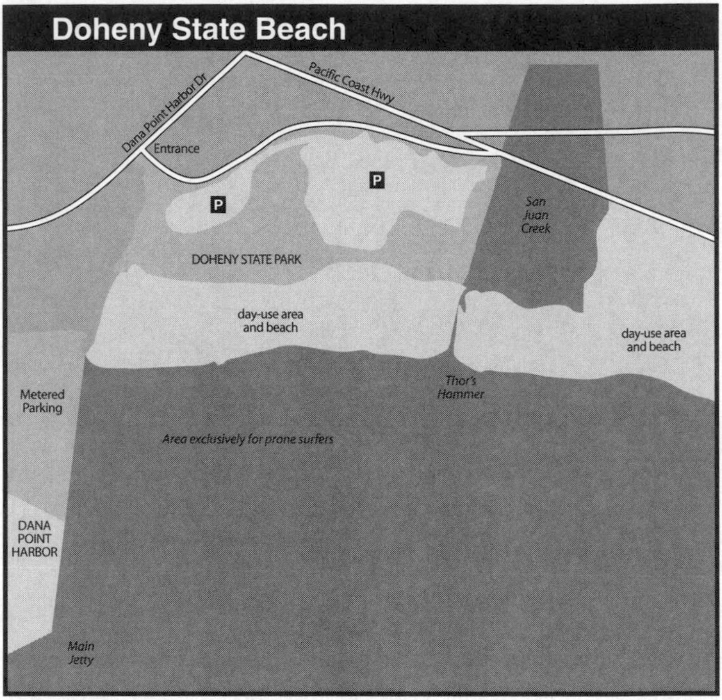

competitors, as well hundreds of others from the stand-up community. It's great fun, but it's not an opportune time for a soulful surf session. On the Friday before the race weekend, it was difficult to find more than a couple feet of open space in the water. (The Battle of the Paddle was moved to Salt Creek Beach Park for 2014. The organizers currently have a five-year contract with the county beach.)

Even without events, crowds can be an issue at Doheny. On warm summer weekends, the surf zone will be littered with boards and bodies. Surfers, particularly longboarders, are still the dominant user group.

Where to Surf SUP boards are allowed only on the lower end of the break, south of the short jetty known as **Thor's Hammer,** which borders the mouth of San Juan Creek. Prone surfers have no such restrictions and will be found, particularly on busy days, from the harbor jetty all the way down to the river mouth.

It's common to find a concentration of surfers just north of Thor's Hammer. This is an ideal takeoff spot for a nice peak that peels beachward and toward the river mouth. I advise against venturing there, though, for several reasons. First of all, you'll get yelled at. The prone surfers all know the rules, and they're more than happy to repeat them. Second, the lifeguards will pull out their speakers and instruct you to move. If you continue to disobey, they have the power to ticket you. Beyond reprobation, there's also the matter of etiquette and fairness. Let the surfers have their waves, give them space, and don't cut them off.

If you're patient and the conditions are right, you have plenty of opportunities to catch waves in the legal SUP zone. For instance, on many days prone surfers and stand-up surfers form a pack offshore of Thor's Hammer, leaving nice peaks to the south uncrowded.

Since my first outing at Doheny, I've had many good days there. I recommend it on many levels. For beginners, the break is fun and forgiving. The waves are slow enough that you need to paddle hard to get into them. The takeoffs are rarely critical, and paddling out through the surf is relatively easy. If you want to learn at Doheny, find a spot south of the jetty, away from the largest pack of surfers. Just concentrate on catching waves, not necessarily catching the best ones. You'll be amazed at how fast you progress.

Even if you aren't a beginner, surfing out of the pack may still be the best option. As you stray south, however, be aware that the break becomes a bit dependent on tide and swell. If the tide is high, the waves tend to break best (and sometimes only) on the reefs outside of Thor's Hammer. Extreme low tides drain the break of almost all its energy. A rising low- to mid-range tide seems to promote the best conditions.

As for swell direction, Doheny really only works on south swells. The jetty and the harbor prevent west swells from wrapping inside. But when the southern hemisphere sends waves our way, Doheny can be a magical spot. With a bit of size, the longboard cruising wave transforms into a fun, carve-able wave. On large swells, the rides can be impossibly long, with section after section almost, but not quite, closing out.

Directions and Parking From I-5, head north on Pacific Coast Highway for 0.8 mile before turning left onto Dana Point Harbor Drive. Turn immediately left into the state park entrance (Park Lantern Drive). If your destination is the metered parking, take the second left. Day use is $15; an annual pass is $195. There is also metered parking at the north end of the beach (don't go into the state park), but this is at the opposite end of the beach from the stand-up zone. Past the entrance kiosk, you'll see the day-use parking on the right. For stand-up surfing, continue to the far end of the parking lot, closest to the creek. It's about 200 yards from the parking lot to the water. Follow the paved path past the grassy picnic area and toward the lifeguard building (it's the only two-story building on the beach). Stay left of the lifeguard building, and launch to the left of the jetty. There is little to no shore break, and the launch is pretty forgiving (except for the stones—see below).

Hazards The beach is fairly rocky, and, particularly at low tide, you'll have to carry your board over some biscuit-sized stones. If you have sensitive feet, you may want to wear booties. Extreme low tide exposes a reef in front of the river mouth and some rocks in front of Thor's Hammer. Generally, however, Doheny is a safe and accessible spot. If you have any questions or concerns, speak with the lifeguards.

Facilities There are outdoor showers, restrooms, a grassy picnic area, covered kiosks, and volleyball courts in the day-use area. There is also camping south of San Juan Creek.

Ability Level Mostly beginner when the surf is small. On large south swells, this break will appeal to all levels of ability.

Break Direction Right.

Crowds You won't ever be alone at Doheny. On summer weekends, the park is chock-full of surfing families. During significant south swells, particularly when other breaks become difficult to manage, Doheny can get very crowded with surfers of all levels and all types. Just about every day, you'll find a crew of regulars—old longboarders who have been surfing the break for longer than anyone can remember.

Tides A rising tide is preferable and best in the low to medium range (1–3 feet or perhaps a bit higher on a big swell).

Best Swell Direction South works best; southwest will work fairly well.

Rules Stand-up surfers are required to stay south of the jetty that borders San Juan Creek.

Water Quality Because of its proximity to San Juan Creek, Doheny Beach often receives some of the lowest grades for water quality. Surfing here after it rains is probably not just unadvisable but dangerous. The good news is that Doheny is generally a summer surf spot that rarely breaks during winter storms.

Local Burrito You've already read my review of **Las Golondrinas** in the profile of Dana Point Harbor and Baby Beach, but this place is so good I just have to mention it twice. Besides burritos, tamales, and tortas, they have an excellent selection of meat, fish, and vegetarian tacos. On Tuesdays, all tacos are half-price—an excellent value that should not be missed. Four out of five economists agree: When you miss Taco Tuesday at Las Golondrinas, you actually lose money. (34069 Doheny Park Road, Capistrano Beach; 949-240-8659, **lasgolondrinas.biz.**)

Los Angeles County

RAT BEACH (See SUP profile on page 110)

MANHATTAN BEACH

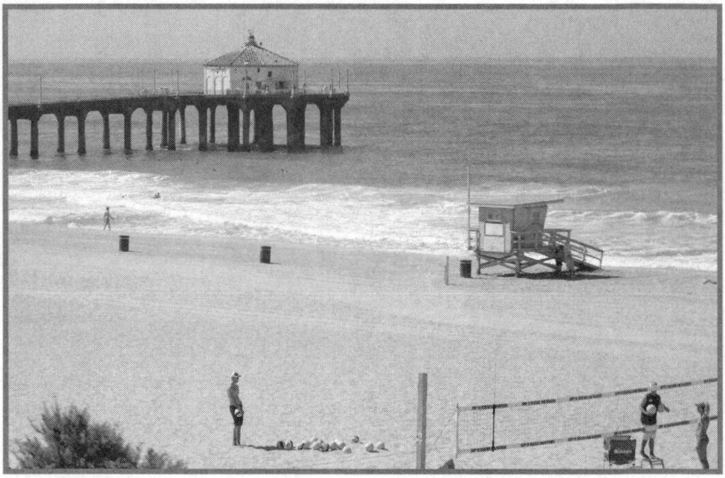

The scene at Manhattan Beach. Bodyboarders and volleyballers dominate the area near the pier.

Overview Manhattan Beach is probably better known for beach volleyball than for surfing. The strand near the pier is covered with nets and courts. On most days, you don't have to look hard to find a few volleyball pros, or at least a few fledging pros, honing their skills on the sand here.

When it comes to water, Manhattan Beach can have fairly consistent surf, particularly in the winter, but the beach break often produces fairly walled conditions. The challenge of surfing Manhattan is finding a workable section, a wave with some shape that doesn't immediately close out. Typically this stretch of coast works best on mixed swells or combined swells—conditions that can produce peaky waves along the sandy shoreline.

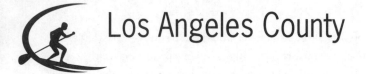

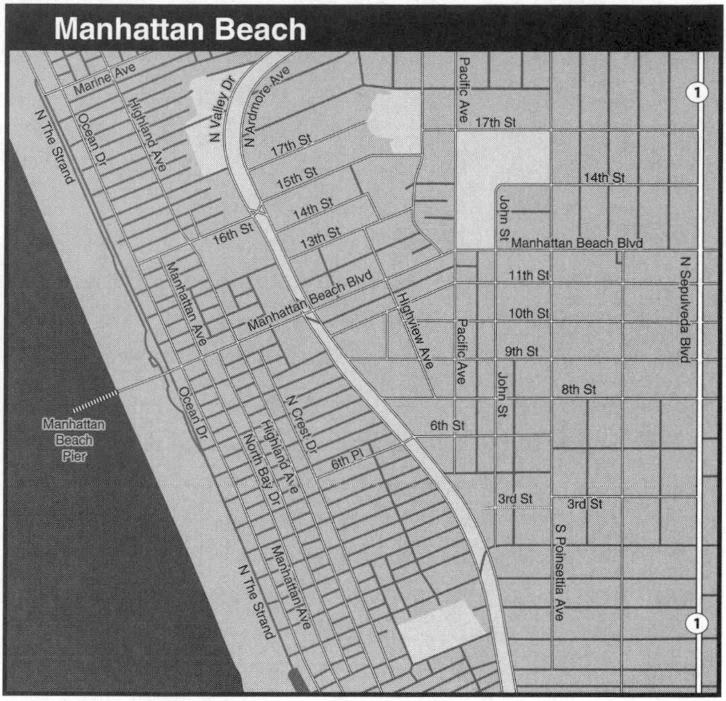

Where to Surf For stand-up surfers, it's probably best to launch north of the pier, then search for an open peak with some semblance of shape and, hopefully, some sort of sandbar that keeps the wave from breaking directly on shore. Obviously, this is not an ideal location for beginners, but it can be a fun spot for intermediate-and-above SUSers (although when the size is large and the shape is poor, the break can be difficult for anyone). At this writing, many local SUSers congregate between **22nd and 26th Streets.** This section of beach has a couple of friendly sand bars that produce peaky waves. Of course this may be subject to change, sand moves, and these particular breaks could shift or change in future years.

Although there is free street parking north of the pier, it isn't always easy to find open spaces. For those not wanting to drive around and hunt, I suggest parking in the pay lot near the pier. Then launch on the north side of the pier and keep paddling up the beach. The pier is at 12th Street and the blocks are short, so the breaks between 22nd and 26th Streets are only about a half-mile north. To get your bearings on the water, you might try lining up near, or just north of, the flagpole at the lifeguard building (on the beach in front of the boardwalk between 22nd and 23rd Streets).

Of course, you can explore other breaks as well, but I advise steering clear of **El Porto,** which is about a mile north of the pier, between 35th and 36th Streets. El Porto attracts a fairly aggressive crew of prone surfers; thus, it won't be the friendliest environment for stand-up surfing.

Directions and Parking From I-405, take the Inglewood exit, then head west on Manhattan Beach Boulevard. Continue 3 miles until you see the pier. Street parking is available on Manhattan Beach Boulevard, along with additional pay lots closer to the sand. Parking costs $1 per hour, payable in 15-minute increments.

Hazards The beach is sandy, and as long as you don't run into the pier, you should be safe. Otherwise, be aware that the waves tend to break fast and close out.

Facilities Bathrooms and outdoor showers near the pier.

Ability Level Intermediate; if the surf is big, definitely advanced. The beach south of the pier will definitely be smaller on south swells.

Break Direction Lefts and rights.

Crowds It's L.A., so there are always people, but Manhattan has a lot of beach and several breaks, so this helps thin out the pack. El Porto on 36th Street tends to be crowded and probably won't be SUS-friendly.

Best Tides Low to medium.

Best Swell Direction It's typically biggest during winter west and northwest swells; the best shape, however, will be found during combination swells (concurrent swells from different directions, conditions that will make the surf peaky).

Water Quality Good. Heal the Bay currently gives Manhattan Beach an A+ rating.

Latigo Point Malibu

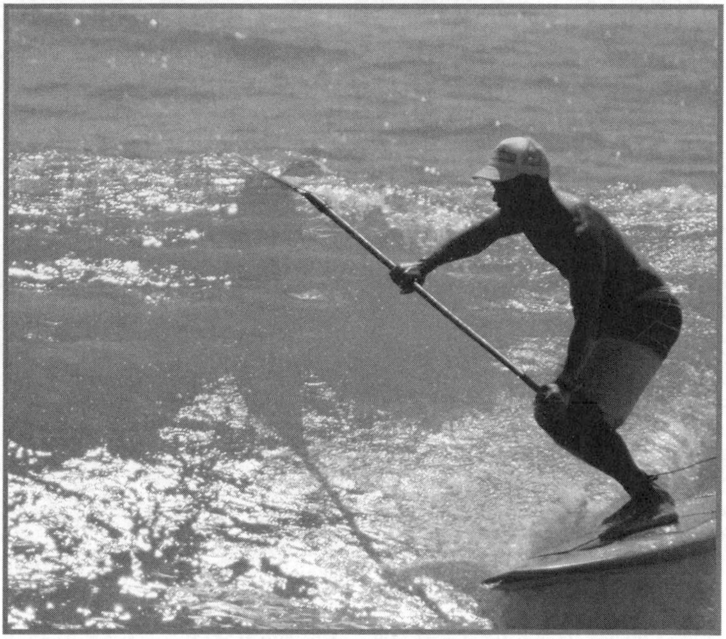

The inside section at Latigo

Overview Surfing in Malibu has a long and storied past. Surfrider Beach, just north of the Malibu pier, may be the mecca of California surfing. Unfortunately, the famous point break suffers from its popularity. On any day with even the slightest bump of surf, Malibu's classic surf spot is packed with boards. Although there are sometimes SUP boards in the mix at Surfrider, it isn't the best spot for stand-up surfing. Don't expect a warm welcome if you head out at Malibu Point with a paddle. Stand-up surfers are better off going to some of the less heralded—and less crowded—breaks along the Malibu coast. Probably the best of these is Latigo Point.

Latigo doesn't break as consistently as Surfrider Beach. It needs about a 3- to 4-foot swell to even work, but large south swells can be

fun here. The wave tends to be a bit mushy and was mostly favored by longboarders before SUP enthusiasts started surfing here. These days it seems to be one of the more established stand-up breaks in Los Angeles. When south swells are pumping, and every surfer in Southern California is eager to get in the water, expect a crowd, but when the surf is smaller, the crowd can be relatively light. Because it doesn't break all the time, surfers tend to forget about Latigo. This is a good thing. For beginning stand-up surfers, a small day here should be easy and friendly—waves slow enough to keep the prone surfers away, but still catchable on the SUP board. On larger days, the wave rolls slowly around the point, allowing for long rides. Latigo holds up and breaks cleanly, even on really large swells, peeling consistently for 100 to 200 yards. Typically, if the point is working, there will also be a beach break farther south and inside the cove—a relatively faster, steeper, and much shorter wave than up at the point.

Where to Surf Paddlers who want to pick off waves closer to shore should be careful of a few exposed rocks just north of the access staircase. The rocks will be either slightly submerged or poking slightly

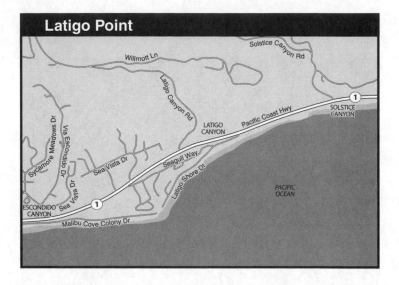

out of the water, depending on the tide. Otherwise, Latigo is fairly user-friendly—a slow but fun wave that can provide some of the longest rides in Malibu. Getting to the beach is relatively easy. Park as close as possible to the access staircase, then head down the short flight to the sandy beach. From the launch it's only about a 10-minute paddle up to the right-breaking point. After a good session, you may be tempted to stop near the Malibu Pier and check out the packed conditions at Surfrider. At this point, you can thank yourself for making the longer drive to Latigo.

Directions and Parking From the Malibu Pier, head 4.8 miles north on Pacific Coast Highway and look for Latigo Canyon Road. Make a U-turn and park on the southbound side of Pacific Coast Highway, either just north or just south of Latigo Shore Drive. There is no public parking on Latigo Shore Drive, but parking is free and legal on the shoulder of PCH. To access the beach, walk to Latigo Shore Drive and look for the brown COASTAL ACCESS sign. Head down the stairs to the beach, then walk up the sand about 50 yards. Launch just to the north of the first set of offshore rocks.

Hazards The rocks near the launch are generally visible and can easily be avoided, but be aware of their presence. There's also a shallow reef inside the point, so check your leash before going out. Otherwise, the break is fairly soft and, except during large south swells, good for less-experienced stand-up surfers.

Facilities None. Just be thankful that there's beach access.

Crowds Generally much less crowded than Malibu, but if the point is working well, it will definitely get busy.

Best Tides Low to medium rising tide. At high tide, depending on the size of the surf, the wave may not break.

Best Swell Direction Southwest, south, and southeast.

Break Direction Right.

Rules There are no limitations on stand-up surfing. The break has the reputation of being friendly for stand-up surfers, but don't assume anything if there's a big crowd.

Water Quality Heal the Bay gives Latigo Beach an A rating for water quality (although there is no sample information for rainy weather). In contrast, several other beaches in Malibu, including Surfrider and Point Dume, consistently receive poor water-quality scores from Heal the Bay.

Other Area Breaks **Sunset Beach,** just south of Gladstones restaurant in Pacific Palisades, is a popular surf spot, and the lower peaks (farther south and around the point) seem to be frequented by stand-up surfers. Both **Point Dume** and **Little Dume** are fairly difficult to access and, on smaller days, would be good for stand-ups. On larger days, however, plenty of surfers will be motivated to make the paddle out to these isolated point breaks. Between North Beach at Leo Carrillo and County Line Beach, there are some fairly uncrowded (again, the isolation factor) beach breaks and reef breaks that would definitely be worth paddling to on a glassy day.

Beach-Access Information The **Los Angeles Urban Rangers** is a group committed to exploring and maintaining public easements along the Malibu coastline. Their two-page PDF beach guide (**tinyurl.com/malibubeachguide**) details every legal entry point along the 27-mile stretch.

Leo Carrillo State Park

(See SUP profile on page 126)

Ventura and Santa Barbara Counties

Mondos

Near Ventura

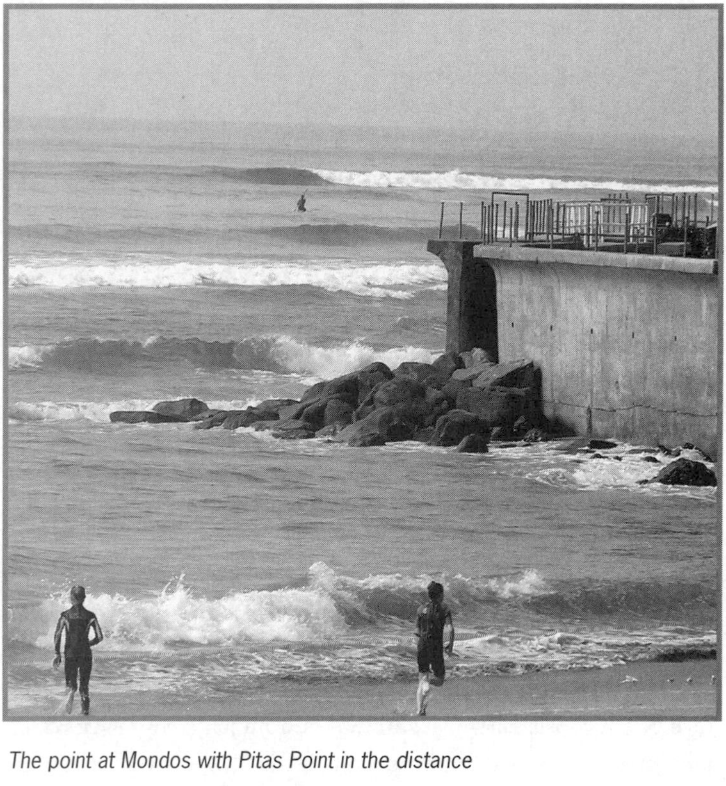

The point at Mondos with Pitas Point in the distance

Overview On the coastal stretch between Ventura and Santa Barbara, there is a remarkable series of point breaks. When winter swells roll down from the Aleutian Islands, these breaks come alive with peeling right-breaking waves. The most heralded of these waves is at Rincon, which is arguably the best point break in California. If Rincon is on, then just about every surfer from Oxnard to Santa Barbara wants to

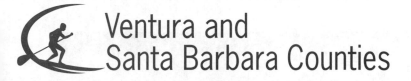

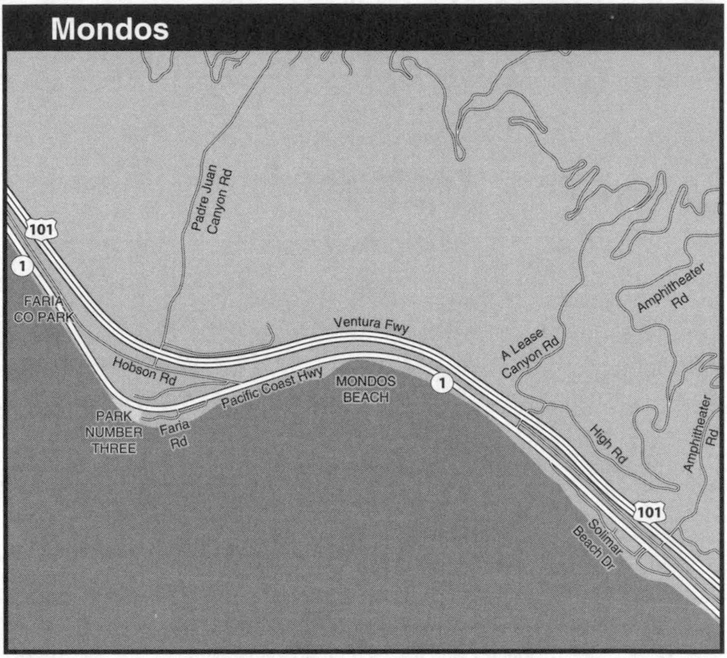

get a piece of it, producing a crowd and a scene not too friendly for stand-up surfers.

Thankfully, there are other nearby points—less heralded and less crowded—that are amenable to stand-up surfing. Of these, Mondos is probably the break with the most consistent crew of stand-up surfers. Mondos will never be confused with Rincon; it's a much slower wave, but it consistently picks up waves from just about every direction. Particularly when the tide is right and northwest swells are pumping, waves wrap nicely around this point, making for long, fun rides.

As you might expect, the prone surfers at Mondos tend to be of the longboard variety. And because the wave tends to roll slowly all the way to the shore, beginning surfers also tend to frequent the break. Depending on the surf size, you have a couple of places to line up: near the submerged reefs just off the point, or a bit farther to the south and slightly inside of the point. The wave closer to the point tends to have a bit more push, and the more accomplished longboarders will surf here. The break south of the point—an easy rolling peak that pushes and re-forms all the way to beach—may be one of the best waves in Southern California for beginner stand-up surfers.

Where to Surf Looking out from the sandy beach, you'll see an immediate point, Mondos, and then Pitas Point, about 500 yards to the north. (Although it can be seen from shore, the wave at Pitas is better viewed from the water than from the beach.) When Mondos is small and not quite working, the waves up at Pitas should have a bit more size and power. It's common to see stand-up surfers make the paddle up to the far point. The uninitiated should be forewarned, though: During significant winter swells, Pitas Point can produce fast, tubing rights that should be left to expert riders.

When there's a decent swell, most stand-up surfers will be content to ride Mondos. The experience here tends to be stress-free, and the vibe in the water is fairly friendly. There isn't much shore break, and the wave tends to wrap close to the point, so the paddle out to the lineup should be relatively easy. Although there are plenty of cobblestones close to the point, much of the shore is smooth and sandy—it's a pretty easy launch. Getting to the water is also fairly easy. Free parking is available on nearby Pacific Coast Highway (park on the shoulder). Although a narrow barrier of boulders separates the highway and the beach, there are a few cut paths that are frequented by surfers. Don't try climbing over the slippery rocks. If you've never been here before, search around a bit to find one of the preferred routes to the beach.

Of course, there are better breaks than Mondos, with waves faster, steeper, and bigger. But I'm not certain that more-challenging waves always provide more fun. A session at Mondos is really what surfing should be about—getting in the water, enjoying the tranquil scenery, and riding a few fun waves. It brings a smile just thinking about it.

Directions and Parking Coming from Ventura on US 101 north, take the State Beaches exit onto CA 1. Continue north for 2.3 miles. The break should be visible once you pass the cluster of homes at Solimar Beach. Parking is free. There is both pull-in and parallel parking along the shoulder of Pacific Coast Highway.

Coming from Santa Barbara on US 101 south, continue past Mussel Shoals and exit at Pacific Coast Highway. Continue south for 3.1 miles, and looked for vehicles with surfboards parked on the left shoulder of the highway.

Best Swell Direction Northwest, west, and southwest.

Best Tides Low to medium. Pitas Point can get fairly hollow at low tide.

Facilities None to speak of, but the beach is quite nice.

OTHER AREA BREAKS

Gold Coast Beach Breaks Between Emma Wood State Beach and Solimar Beach, Pacific Coast Highway fronts a long and narrow swath of coastline. There are no established and consistent breaks here, but under the right conditions—a medium tide and a mixed swell—there may be an opportunity to find some fun peaks along this stretch. When other area breaks are crowded, this wide-open section of beach may offer a chance to find a wave of one's own.

C-Street Also known as Surfer's Point, this flat, rounded headland just north of the Ventura Pier produces a series of right-breaking waves. At the top of the point is the most aggressive and most crowded of the breaks. Farther inside, and closer to the pier, the wave tends to roll more. Stand-up surfers tend to launch at the south end of the main parking lot, then paddle south toward the pier. On large west and northwest swells, this wave wraps and wraps around the point, allowing for long, super-fun rides. Parking in the lot runs $2 per day, and there is free surf-check parking on the street (up to 24 minutes).

Hobson County Park The park is roughly 4 miles north of Mondos on Pacific Coast Highway. There isn't much of a beach here, but there are a few peaky waves that wrap around the curved rocky shore. Day-use parking is limited but free.

Santa Barbara Beaches

See page 137 for information on Leadbetter Beach and page 140 for information on Goleta Beach and Campus Point.

Santa Barbara North

See page 144 for information on Refugio State Beach and page 146 for information on El Capitán State Beach.

Post–surfing session happiness

Photo courtesy of Izzy Tihanyi/Surf Diva

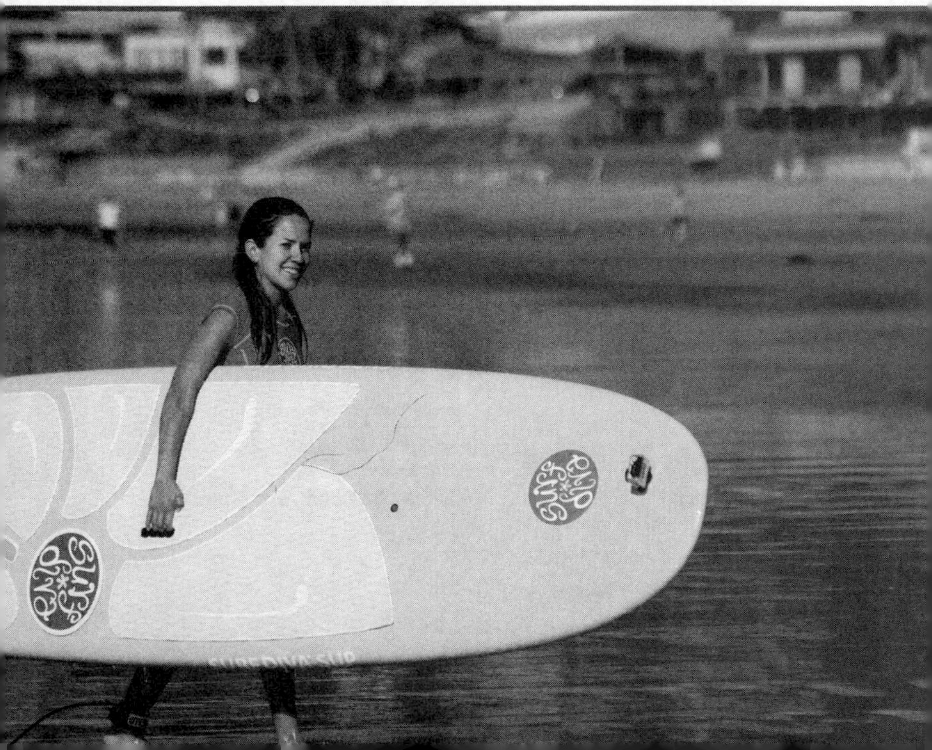

Appendix 1: SUP Shops

San Diego County

Carlsbad

LEGENDS SUP
2658 State St.
Carlsbad, CA 92008
800-515-4863, **legendssup.com**

La Jolla

MITCH'S SURF SHOP
631 Pearl St.
La Jolla, CA 92037
858-459-5933
mitchssurfshop.com

SURF DIVA
2160 Avenida de la Playa
La Jolla, CA 92660
858-454-8273, **surfdiva.com**

Leucadia

PADDLE PLANET
996 N. Coast Highway, Ste. A
Leucadia, CA 92024
760-602-9767, **paddleplanet.net**

National City

ISLE SURF SHOP
340 W. 26th St., Ste. E
National City, CA 91950
888-569-7873, **islesurfboards.com**

Point Loma

OEX POINT LOMA
5060 N. Harbor Dr., Ste. 165
Point Loma, CA 92106
619-224-4241, **oexpointloma.com**

San Diego

CREED SUP
1085 Bay Blvd.
San Diego, CA 91911
619-821-8200, **creedsup.com**

TOWER PADDLE BOARDS
845 Garnet Ave.
San Diego, CA 92109
866-622-4477
towerpaddleboards.com

WEST COAST PADDLE SPORTS
4360 Morena Blvd., Ste. 130
San Diego, CA 92117
858-272-3278
westcoastpaddlesports.com

YOLO BOARD SAN DIEGO
1055 Rosecrans St.
San Diego, CA 92106
619-574-6991
yoloboard.com/yolo-board-san-diego

Solana Beach

JOE BLAIR SURF
365 N. Highway 101
(behind Mitch's Surf Shop)
Solana Beach, CA 92075
760-809-9074
jblairsurf.com/sup/sup-boards

Orange County

Corona Del Mar

HOBIE SURF SHOP
3140 E. Coast Highway
Corona Del Mar, CA 92625
949-706-8090, **hobiesurfshop.com**

SUP TO YOU
1648 Newport Blvd., Ste. A
Corona Del Mar, CA 92627
949-715-7300; **sup-to-you.com**

Costa Mesa

PADDLE SURF WAREHOUSE
629 Terminal Way, Ste. 26
Costa Mesa, CA 92627
949-574-5897
paddlesurfwarehouse.com

Dana Point

HOBIE SURF SHOP
34174 Pacific Coast Highway
Dana Point, CA 92629
949-496-2366, **hobiesurfshop.com**

INFINITY SURFBOARD COMPANY
24382 Del Prado Ave.
Dana Point, CA 92629
949-661-6699
infinitysurf.com/sup

Huntington Beach

REI HUNTINGTON BEACH
7777 Edinger Ave., Ste. 138
Huntington Beach, CA 92647
714-379-1938
rei.com/stores/huntington-beach

SUP-POSITION
15571 Commerce Lane
Huntington Beach, CA 92649
714-899-3020, **sup-position.com**

Laguna Beach

BRAWNER BOARDS
1130 S. Coast Highway
Laguna Beach, CA 92651
949-715-9730
brawnerboards.com

CA SURF N' PADDLE
(at Costa Azul Surf Shop)
695 S. Coast Highway
Laguna Beach, CA 92651
949-497-1423
casurfshop.com

HOBIE SURF SHOP
294 Forest Ave.
Laguna Beach, CA 92651
949-497-3304, **hobiesurfshop.com**

SUP TO YOU
2097-A Laguna Canyon Rd.
Laguna Beach, CA 92651
949-715-7300, **suptoyou.com**

Newport Beach

PADDLE POWER
1500 W. Balboa Blvd., Ste. 101
Newport Beach, CA 92663
949-675-1215
paddlepowerh2o.com

San Clemente

TRY STAND UP PADDLE
844-787-7873, **trystandup.com**

Tustin

REI TUSTIN
2962 El Camino Real
Tustin, CA 92782
714-505-020
rei.com/stores/tustin

San Pedro

CAPTAIN KIRK'S
525 N. Harbor Blvd.
San Pedro, CA 90731
310-833-3397
captainkirks.com

Los Angeles County

Hermosa Beach

TARSAN SUP
936 Hermosa Ave.
Hermosa Beach, CA 90254
310-798-7878, **tarsanstandup.com**

Manhattan Beach

REI MANHATTAN BEACH
1800 Rosecrans Ave., Ste. E
Manhattan Beach, CA 90266
310-727-0728
rei.com/stores/manhattan-beach

Marina Del Rey

ACTION WATER SPORTS
4144 Lincoln Blvd.
Marina Del Rey, CA 90291
310-627-2233
actionwatersports.com

PRO SUP SHOP
4175 Admiralty Way
Marina Del Rey, CA 90292
310-945-8450; **prosupshop.com**

Redondo Beach

TARSAN SUP
831 N. Harbor Drive
Redondo Beach, CA 90277
310-798-2200, **tarsanstandup.com**

XSTREAMLINE PADDLESPORTS
1861 N. Gaffey St., Ste. I
San Pedro, CA 90731
310-514-9514
xstreamline.com

Santa Monica

POSEIDON PADDLE AND SURF
1654 Ocean Ave.
Santa Monica, CA 90401
310-694-8428
poseidonstandup.com

REI SANTA MONICA
402 Santa Monica Blvd.
Santa Monica, CA 90401
310-458-4370
rei.com/stores/santa-monica

Torrance

OLYMPUS BOARD SHOP
4807 Torrance Blvd.
Torrance, CA 90503
310-214-1800
olympusboardshop.net

Camarillo

PADDLESURF OUTLET
396 Ventura Blvd.
Camarillo, CA 93010
805-415-7674
paddlesurfoutlet.com

Santa Barbara

BLUELINE STAND UP PADDLE SURF
24 E. Mason St.
Santa Barbara, CA 93101
805-845-5606
bluelinepaddlesurf.com

SUP SPORTS
121 Santa Barbara St.
Santa Barbara, CA 93101
888-805-9978 or 805-962-7877
supsports.com

Appendix 2: Locations for Rentals and Lessons

San Diego County

Carlsbad

2 STAND UP GUYS
4509 Adams St.
Carlsbad, CA 92008
347-489-3926, **2standupguys.com**

Coronado

SUP CORONADO
(Meets at Coronado Tidelands Park, 2000 Mullinex Drive)
619-888-7686, **supcoronado.com**

La Jolla

SURF DIVA
2160 Avenida de la Playa
La Jolla, CA 92660
858-454 -8273, **surfdiva.com**

Mission Bay

BLISS PADDLE YOGA
858-215-3661
paddleboardbliss.com

MISSION BAY AQUATIC CENTER
1001 Santa Clara Place
San Diego, CA 92109
858-488-1000
mbaquaticcenter.com

MISSION BAY SPORTCENTER
1010 Santa Clara Place
San Diego, CA 92109
858-488-1004
missionbaysportcenter.com

OEX MISSION BAY
1010 Santa Clara Place
Mission Bay, CA 92109
619-866-6129, **oexmissionbay.com**

SAN DIEGO PADDLE COMPANY
Shelter Island Dr.
San Diego, CA 92106
619-786-5782
facebook.com/sandiegokayakrentals

Oceanside

BOAT RENTALS OF AMERICA
256 Harbor Drive S.
Oceanside, CA 92054
760-722-0028, **boats4rent.com**

San Diego

ALOHA STAND UP PADDLE
760-213-4133
alohastanduppaddle.com

PADDLE INTO FITNESS
paddleintofitness.com

SAN DIEGO EXCELLENT ADVENTURES
619-962-9306, **getwetsandiego.com**

SAN DIEGO SURFING SCHOOL
4850 Cass St.
San Diego, CA 92109
858-205-7683
sandiegosurfingschool.com

THE SUP CONNECTION
2592 Laning Rd.
San Diego, CA 92106
619-365-4225
sandiegosuprentals.com

SURFER GIRLS
4500 Ocean Blvd.
San Diego, CA 92109
858-205-7683, **alohasurfergirls.com**

Solana Beach

MITCH'S SURF SHOP
363 N. Highway 101
Solana Beach, CA 92075
858-481-1354
mitchssurfshop.com

Orange County

Dana Point

PADDLE SURF WAREHOUSE
24682 Del Prado
Dana Point, CA 92629
949-488-8041
paddlesurfwarehouse.com

WESTWIND SAILING
34451 Ensenada Place
(Baby Beach, Dana Point Harbor)
949-923-2215
westwindsailing.com

Laguna Beach

BLISS PADDLE YOGA
949-529-4242
paddleboardbliss.com

BRAWNER BOARDS
1130 S. Coast Highway
Laguna Beach, CA 92651
949-715-9730, **brawnerboards.com**

CA SURF N' PADDLE
(at Costa Azul Surf Shop)
695 S. Coast Highway
Laguna Beach, CA 92651
949-497-1423
casurfshop.com

LA VIDA LAGUNA
1257 S. Coast Highway
Laguna Beach, CA 92651
949-275-7511
lavidalaguna.com

Newport Beach

NEWPORT AQUATIC CENTER
1 White Cliffs Drive
Newport Beach, CA 92660
949-626-7725
newportaquaticcenter.com

PADDLE POWER
1500 W. Balboa Blvd., Ste.101
Newport Beach, CA 92663
949-675-1215
paddlepowerh2o.com

San Clemente

BRAWNER BOARDS
220 Avenida Vaquero
San Clemente, CA 92672
949-429-9601
brawnerboards.com

Sunset Beach

OEX SUNSET BEACH
16910 Pacific Coast Highway
Sunset Beach, CA 90742
562-592-6080
oexsunsetbeach.com

Los Angeles County

Long Beach/Belmont Shore

LONG BEACH AQUATICS CENTER
5411 E. Ocean Blvd.
Long Beach, CA 90803
562-434-0999

Malibu

MALIBU SURF SHACK
22935 Pacific Coast Hwy.
Malibu, CA 90265
310-456-8508
malibusurfshack.com

RADFISH MALIBU
310-433-1767, **radfishmalibu.com**

Manhattan Beach

NIKAU KAI WATERMAN SHOP
1300 Highland Ave.
Manhattan Beach, CA 90266
310-545-7007, **nikaukai.com**

Marina Del Rey

PADDLE METHOD
14110 Palowan Way
Marina Del Rey, CA 90292
310-770-7291; **paddlemethod.com**

PRO SUP SHOP
4175 Admiralty Way
Marina Del Rey, CA 90292
310-945-8350, **prosupshop.com**

Redondo Beach

TARSAN SUP
831 N. Harbor Drive
Redondo Beach, CA 90277
310-798-2200, **tarsanstandup.com**

San Pedro

XSTREAMLINE PADDLESPORTS
1861 N. Gaffey St., Ste. I
San Pedro, CA 90731
310-514-9514, **xstreamline.com**

Santa Monica

POSEIDON PADDLE AND SURF
1654 Ocean Ave.
Santa Monica, CA 90401
310-694-8428
poseidonstandup.com

Ventura and Santa Barbara Counties

Santa Barbara

CHANNEL ISLANDS OUTFITTERS PADDLE SPORTS CENTER
Locations at Santa Barbara Harbor (117-B Harbor Way, Santa Barbara, CA 93019) and Goleta Beach (5986 Sandspit Road, Goleta, CA 93117).
805–617-3425, **paddlesportsca.com**

SANTA BARBARA SAILING CENTER
Santa Barbara Harbor, next to the boat ramp
805-962-2826, **sbsail.com**

SUP SPORTS
121 Santa Barbara St.
Santa Barbara, CA 93101
888-805-9978 or 805-962-7877
supsports.com

Ventura

PADDLESURF OUTLET
Lessons and rentals available at Ventura Harbor and Channel Islands Harbor; see URL below for directions.
805-415-7674
paddlesurfoutlet.com/id2.html

Appendix 3: A Month-by-Month Guide to Paddleboard Events in Southern California

January

HANOHANO HUKI OCEAN CHALLENGE Demonstrating goodwill across the paddling community, this fun race through San Diego's Mission Bay includes classes for SUPers, outriggers, surf skiers, and prone paddlers. It may not be an elite race, but it attracts massive group of paddlers. Details: **hanohano.com/events.**

February

LANAKILA CLASSIC Sponsored by a Redondo Beach outrigger paddling club, this event takes place in Seaside Lagoon, just south of King's Harbor in Redondo Beach). The race features a short course and a long course as well as several divisions for SUP competitors. Details: **paddleguru.com/races/lanakilaclassic2015.**

March

ADLER PADDLER Part race and part fun paddle, this event is designed to raise awareness about thoracic aortic dissection—the genetic heart defect that killed the event's namesake, Steve Adler, as well as actor John Ritter. Proceeds from the event help fund The John Ritter Foundation. Details: **paddlewithpurpose.wordpress.com, johnritterfoundation.org.**

MICKEY MUÑOZ MONGOOSE CUP Surf legend Mickey Muñoz promotes this race to raise funds and awareness for the Wounded Warrior Project. Taking place at Baby Beach in Dana Point Harbor, the event is open to paddlers of all abilities. There are also instructional clinics for new paddlers. Details: **tinyurl.com/mongoosecup.**

May

MALIBU DOWNWINDER Since 2004, this point-to-point race has sought to take advantage of the strong springtime winds along the Malibu coast. Beginning at Point Mugu, racers head downwind for 7 miles to Leo Carrillo State Park, where an awards ceremony and beach barbecue await. Details: **malibudw.blogspot.com.**

June

SANTA MONICA PADDLEBOARD RACE AND OCEAN FESTIVAL This event honors a tradition of paddleboard races in Santa Monica that dates back to the 1930s. Both the long course and the short, fun course have divisions ranging from Surfboard Class to Elite Men and Women. Details: **santamonicapier.org/pier-paddle.**

September

WATER WARRIOR BEACH FESTIVAL Held at Camp Pendleton, the 5K and 10K paddling races include flat-water paddling, open-ocean paddling, and a beach run. If that weren't enough, there's also something called the Amphibious Assault Race, where paddlers are required to navigate through obstacles on and off the water. Details: **mccscp.com/waterwarrior.**

October

BATTLE OF THE PADDLE This is the big prize for Southern California stand-up paddling. The BOP is a phenomenon that attracts heaps of vendors, competitors, and spectators. Although the surf-intensive format might dissuade beginning paddlers, surfboard-class heats are offered for all ages. (The race used to be held in September, but starting in 2015 the date has been changed to October.) Details: **battleofthepaddle.com.**

November

SDOCC LA JOLLA SHORES INVITATIONAL Another outrigger-sponsored event, this race in beautiful La Jolla now features a 6.5-mile course exclusively for SUPers. Details: **tinyurl.com/lajollashoresinvitational.** The website lists information for the 2014 race, but you should be able to find out more closer to the 2015 event; plus, the website has e-mail contacts for the organizers (click "Contact Race").

December

BECKY STUART MEMORIAL RACE This is a great community event hosted by the Oceanside Outrigger Canoe Club. Following the 4-mile and 8-mile races, a homemade lunch of chili and potatoes is served. The race begins at Dolphin Dock on the west side of Oceanside Harbor, heads out into the ocean, and finishes inside the harbor. Details: **tinyurl.com/beckystuartmemorialrace.** As with the La Jolla Shores Invitational, the website lists information for the 2014 race but includes e-mail contacts (click "Contact Race").

Index

Page references followed by *fig* indicate an illustrated figure or a photograph; followed by *m* indicates a map.

About the Author

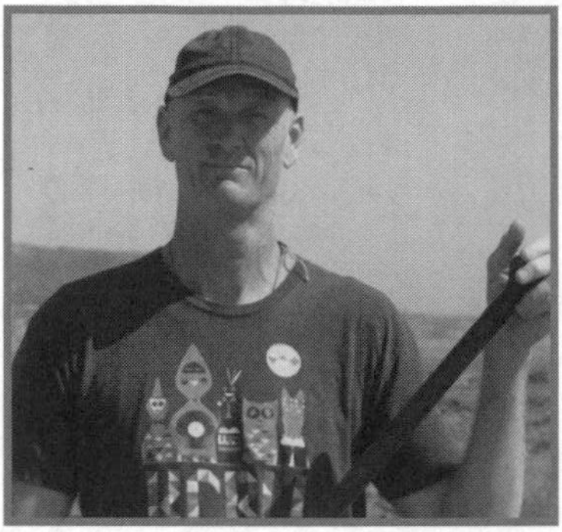

Photo: Logan Schoembs

DAVID WOMACK IS a California native and a longtime Laguna Beach resident. As a child, many years before stand-up paddleboards were invented, he spent his summers bodysurfing at El Morro Beach (now Crystal Cove State Park). These days he can often be found paddling around the reefs of Laguna Beach and the stand-up-surfing waves of south Orange County.

David received his MFA in creative writing in 2005 from UC Riverside, where he wrote about things that had nothing to do with paddling and ocean sports. He is also an avid windsurfer and enthusiastic mountain biker, and sometimes he becomes preoccupied with puzzles. His first book, *Mountain Bike! Orange County,* was published by Menasha Ridge Press in 2007. His writing also has appeared in *Littoral* magazine and online at **connotationpress.com** and **fiction365.com.**